W9-BZY-048

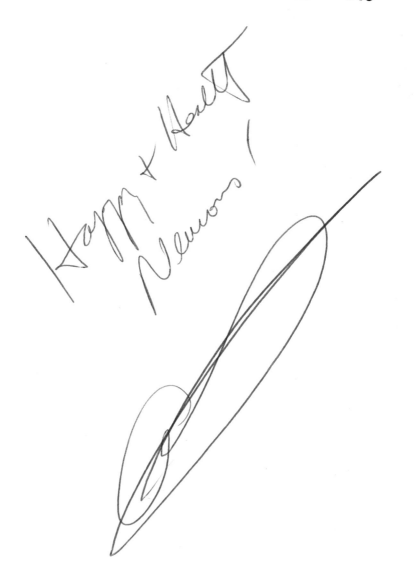

# THE BRAIN
# WELLNESS
# PLAN

# THE BRAIN
# WELLNESS
# PLAN

## BREAKTHROUGH MEDICAL, NUTRITIONAL, AND IMMUNE-BOOSTING THERAPIES

### Dr. Jay Lombard,
**Board Certified Neurologist**
### and Carl Germano, RD, CNS, LDN

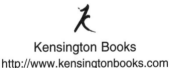

Kensington Books
http://www.kensingtonbooks.com

KENSINGTON BOOKS are published by

Kensington Publishing Corp.
850 Third Avenue
New York, NY 10022

Copyright © 1997 by Dr. Jay Lombard and Carl Germano

Library of Congress Card Catalog Number: 97-072050
ISBN 1-57566-230-2

First Kensington Hardcover Printing: August, 1997
10  9  8  7  6  5  4  3  2  1

Printed in the United States of America

This book is dedicated to my wife, Rita, for her endless devotion and love, and to my parents for teaching me that intellectual curiosity must always be coupled with compassion.

—Jay Lombard

To my wife, Alise, for her inexhaustible love and patience. To my son, Grant, and daughter, Samantha, who give special meaning and cohesion to my life. Lastly, to my mother, Frances, for the wealth of love and support she has provided me. All of you mean the world to me.

—Carl Germano

# ACKNOWLEDGMENTS

Thanks to Holly Robinson for her incredible intelligence and guidance in writing this book; to Jerry Hickey for introducing me to Carl Germano; to the physicians and teachers—Dr. Rudolph Nisi, Dr. Steven Bock, Dr. Kenneth Bock, Dr. Leo Galland, and Dr. Steven Kraskow—who teach by example the sacredness of healing and that a patient's well-being is always of primary importance; and finally, to the countless researchers who have devoted their lives to solving the mystery of disease in the hope of alleviating those who are suffering.

—Jay Lombard

Special thanks to Rand Skolnick for providing me the opportunity to "shine" and work for the supplement company that continues to set the standards for the industry; to Jerry Hickey for bringing Dr. Lombard and me together to complete this important work; to Holly Robinson (and her fax machine), whose touch is felt on every page; to photographer Jill LeVine, for making me look good; to Lee Heiman, for his continued support and valued suggestions; to Tracy Bernstein, for her editing of the manuscript; to Paul Dinas, for working to accommodate my anxiety of getting this book published as quickly as possible; and to Kensington Publishing, for believing in this important work. Most importantly, thanks to all the researchers, nutritional scientists, and physicians who sought to better understand the true meaning of clinical nutrition and functional medicine above and beyond what the establishment led them to believe. Lastly, to the pioneers of progressive nutritional supplementation for the prevention and treatment of disease, I thank you all for your commitment and significant contributions to the field of nutritional medicine.

—Carl Germano

# CONTENTS

# INTRODUCTION

For too many of us, the prospect of aging is shadowed by gloomy stereotypes. Perhaps we imagine an elderly man who can scarcely maintain his balance as he shuffles outside to retrieve the morning paper, or an older woman so forgetful that she can no longer name her own children, much less drive to the grocery store.

As we age, all of us lose brain cells as a result of genetic weaknesses, infections, injuries, and environmental toxins—the combination of which often leads to brain disease and dysfunction.

And the brain—our body's most complex organ, despite its compact three-pound size—commands everything from memory to sex drive. So it is little wonder that many of us have accepted the notion that we are fated to suffer neurological illnesses and lose brain power as we age.

Thankfully, those days are over. New investigations conducted by top researchers worldwide have led today's most informed health care practitioners to this promising conclusion: No matter how old you are, keeping your brain healthy is the key to living at your fullest, most vital capacity.

In *The Brain Wellness Plan,* you will find valuable insights and the most current medical information available about brain health. In addition to offering a practical, two-step "Brain Wellness Plan" for preventing brain disease and boosting brain power through optimum nutrition, this book provides complete treatment protocols for the most common neurological illnesses affecting Americans today.

These protocols—aimed at effectively treating Alzheimer's, Parkinson's, multiple sclerosis, ALS, ADHD, chronic fatigue syndrome, and depression—represent the first of their kind in complementary medicine, integrating breakthrough advances in nutrition with medical and immune-boosting therapies. As such, they highlight how well we can now harness nature in our efforts to prevent and heal brain disease.

Our combined clinical, teaching, and research experience— as a chief neurologist at a New York medical center and private practitioner in neurology and neuropsychiatry, and as a certified nutritionist with nearly two decades of clinical practice and ten years invested in research—has taught us that employing innovative, complementary medicine techniques in preventing and treating neurological illnesses is the best road to brain health.

Our overarching goal in writing *The Brain Wellness Plan* is to give you the tools—and the inspiration—to make informed choices when caring for yourself or someone you love. Join us, and become your own—and your family's—best advocate in maintaining and restoring brain health.

## The First Secret to Keeping Our Brains Well: A Healthy Brain-Immune Connection

Thanks to well-documented scientific studies conducted at prestigious medical centers around the world, today we can describe in detail the intricate dance between the brain and the immune system, the brain's most important partner in health.

In the first section of this book, we invite you to fully explore the partnership between the brain and the immune system, and to learn how these two seemingly disparate body systems work as one in health and disease.

The dawning appreciation among health care practitioners of the brain's role as a dynamic organ working in concert with other body systems means that you can now harvest information from the front lines of medicine to maintain optimum health.

In *The Brain Wellness Plan,* you will read about neurotransmitters, the brain's chemical messengers so vital to your well-being. Some of the key neurotransmitters we discuss are media superstars like serotonin and dopamine, whose roles have already been well documented. We also introduce certain understudies ready to steal the limelight. These include neurotransmitters like nitric oxide, a gas whose multiple functions in the brain-immune connection we are just beginning to recognize.

In describing the immune system, we will talk about the newly recognized role of immunotransmitters, the chemical messengers of the immune system, in keeping your body healthy. *The Brain Wellness Plan* then guides you through the latest scientific evidence describing the consequences of disturbing the delicate brain-immune balance. We fully discuss the link between various neurological illnesses and genetic factors, toxins, stress, and infections. In addition, you will discover why the brain is so vulnerable to attack by your own body's immune system—and what you can do to prevent it.

## Nutritional Therapies with the Power to Heal

Nutritional science is barely more than a century old. Yet, we have already reaped astounding answers to the most essential questions about how the foods we eat have the power to help us live longer, healthier lives.

From the B vitamins to ginkgo biloba, some nutritional compounds can profoundly influence all aspects of brain and immune function. In *The Brain Wellness Plan,* we present the results of significant basic research and detail clinical trials documenting specific ways in which these nutritional agents maintain brain health and reverse neurological diseases.

In our two-step plan to brain health, we offer a guide to nutrients with proven potential in promoting the health of your gastrointestinal tract, allowing for better absorption of essential brain-strengthening nutrients, and a comprehensive list of foods and supplements you can start incorporating into your diet immediately to support your overall health.

## What About Brain Nutrients?

Besides taking steps to ensure your overall well-being, you can also begin now—no matter what your age—to add the nutrients so essential to supporting brain health and a vital brain-immune connection.

*The Brain Wellness Plan* provides a comprehensive discussion of "neuroimmunomodulation," the exciting concept of using specific nutrients tailored to smooth the essential two-way chemical dialogue between the brain and the immune system.

After introducing basic neuroimmunomodulators that serve as the foundations for brain health, such as the powerful new generation of brain-protecting antioxidants, we move into Part II of the book. From Alzheimer's to multiple sclerosis, from Lou Gehrig's disease to depression, we devote the entire second section to a detailed discussion of seven common neurological illnesses.

Besides offering you an overview of each disease and its impact on the brain, we present practical ways to ascertain that you or your loved one has received the most accurate, sophisticated diagnosis possible, followed by a complete, disease-specific blueprint for care, which lists:

1. Recommended dosages of safe, effective nutritional agents you can take immediately to treat that particular neurological disorder, and
2. How to work with your health care provider to incorporate cutting-edge medications and hormonal therapies into a complete disease treatment plan.

Here, you will discover evidence for just how neuroimmunomodulating therapies have proven beneficial in both successfully preventing the root causes of disease and in treating clinical symptoms.

Restoring the deficiency of dopamine associated with Parkinson's disease, for example, is a key step in improving motor functions and balance. We also recommend nutritional agents that serve to protect neurons from further damage and destruction.

In treating Alzheimer's, we focus on nutrients that improve blood flow, provide adequate fuel for cells, and preserve neurons that synthesize and release acetylcholine, the memory neurotransmitter. And for multiple sclerosis patients, we recommend a diet low in saturated fat and high in the omega-3 fatty acids so essential in rebuilding myelin, the nerve cell sheaths, and in modulating the immune system's inflammatory responses.

Finally, at the end of the book, we provide a reference guide listing alternative medical information resources and support groups, and an appendix of notes chronicling the scientific studies supporting the information you will find here.

## Become a Partner in Building a Better Brain-Immune Connection

Millions of people are affected by the ravages of brain injuries each year. Until recently, neurological diseases were considered irreversible and permanent, and to this day some physicians feel they have nothing to offer in terms of healing them.

Now, armed with new understanding of the biochemical processes involved in the brain-immune connection and ways to modulate those processes, you no longer have to accept the idea that brain disease or dysfunction is inevitable with age. Instead, you can work with your health care practitioners to aggressively prevent neurological disorders and to restore brain health should they occur.

Our ability to maintain brain wellness and to heal ourselves rests on our ability to educate ourselves about the underlying causes of disease, and on our determination to fight back with knowledge. We hope you will use this book as your first step toward preventing and reversing brain disease—and take advantage of this marvelous medical revolution to make the most of your life.

## PART I

# The Brain-Immune Connection

# BRAIN-IMMUNE CONNECTION BASICS

From the earliest moment of development to the last stages of your life, your brain and immune system are involved in a constant, ever-changing dialogue. Each influences the other in specific and profound ways.

The growth of the human brain and its health are dependent on proper immune function from infancy. Conversely, the premature demise of brain cells in diseases such as Alzheimer's, Parkinson's, and ALS is linked to immune system breakdown.

Biological communication between your body's many systems relies on messenger molecules which travel between cells and act in concert with one another. In this chapter, you will learn about the ongoing chemical dialogue between the brain and the immune system, a connection that depends on two languages: the neurotransmitters of the brain, and the immunotransmitters of the immune system.

First, though, let's take a look at the regional control center for monitoring this vital biological dialogue, a brain structure known as the hypothalamus.

## The Hypothalamus: Where Brain and Immune System Meet

The hypothalamus is an area of the brain no larger than a pea, yet its complex communication pathways connect your brain with your endocrine, cardiovascular, and immune systems. Like a master conductor in a biological symphony, the hypothalamus orchestrates the production and release of thyroid, stress, growth, and sex hormones. It also controls the amount of insulin released by the pancreas.

Furthermore, this tiny brain structure links our emotions to our bodily responses. For instance, anger, depression, and anxiety are all mediated by chemical communication signals that originate in the hypothalamus. These signals include neurotransmitters and substances known as "hormone-releasing factors," or neuropeptides—protein-like substances which regulate body temperature, level of alertness, blood pressure, respiratory rate, appetite, and reproductive functions.

Now, in addition to commanding this vast spectrum of responses, recent scientific discoveries have linked the hypothalamus to immune function as well. Research has demonstrated that this part of the brain exchanges a significant amount of information with the body's immune system via their respective neurotransmitters and immunotransmitters.

Hypothalamic messengers allow the brain to directly influence the immune system and either increase or decrease its activity. The immune system even has receptor sites for these neurotransmitters. The receptor sites are found on white blood cells, lymph nodes, and various other immune organs.

Conversely, the brain's hypothalamus is directly and continuously influenced by the immune system. Certain brain regions are specifically designed to receive immunotransmitters, and in this way the immune system can profoundly influence brain metabolism, the electrical activity of neurons, and the synthesis and release of neurotransmitters.

This elaborate biological communication network, which we refer to as the brain-immune connection, is the basis of your well-being or your vulnerability to a particular disease. As you will see throughout *The Brain Wellness Plan*, your health depends on the ongoing ability of the brain and the immune system to communicate effectively in both directions.

## Neurons: Speaking the Brain's Language

When mystery novelist Agatha Christie's favorite detective, Hercule Poirot, is up against a tough case to solve, he often looks for answers in "the little grey cells." Those little grey cells are the neurons in our brains.

*Neuron,* the word for the brain's most basic cellular unit, is Greek for "string." Indeed, people during the Greek and Roman eras drew a parallel between man, who is manipulated by the gods, and puppets on strings. However, even early on, physicians such as Hippocrates (*ca.* 460–377 B.C.) managed to persuade at least some in the scientific community that diseases were not punishments from the gods, but the result of natural causes.

Today, we are able to use tools such as digitized computer microscope systems to actually see what is happening in the brain, leading us to understand a great deal about brain function and to closely map specific disease pathways.

Essentially, the brain relies on efficient connections between neighboring neurons to process information it receives from sense organs such as your eyes, ears, and skin, as well as from within your body. That way, your brain can keep track of what's going on in your body's external and internal environments and instruct other bodily systems to respond accordingly.

Your emotional and physical health depends on how well your brain cells communicate with one another—and with the rest of your body—via neurotransmitters.

## The Brain's Messengers

Neurotransmitters are the brain's pony express messengers, chemicals that leap across the tiny gaps, or synapses, between brain cells. If there is a match between the neurotransmitter's password and the chemical gates of the receptors of the receiving cell, the event causes the receiving neuron to either fire or shut down, depending on the message received.

In other words, each of your neurons has certain receptors on their cell surfaces, which we call membranes, and these receptors act as receiving platforms for messages from various neurotransmitters. This exacting process requires a specific match between the receptor and the neurotransmitter, much as every lock requires a specific key.

Once a specific neurotransmitter binds to a neuron receptor, it sets a chain reaction into motion within the cell. These chemical reactions in turn then regulate and control every cellular process, producing specific biological effects.

Receptors found in neuron membranes are highly specialized in terms of their structure, and that structure is dependent upon the condition of the cell membrane. The cell membrane, which is composed mostly of proteins and lipids, is in a constant state of flux. Changes in cell membranes actually occur from moment to moment, and are uniquely affected by factors such as the emotions, diet, and the immune system. Even slight alterations in this specialized cell membrane design can have negative consequences on the ability of neurotransmitters to produce the desired effects, and can ultimately cause disease.

For example, patients with Alzheimer's suffer massive destruction of the brain cells that release a memory-enhancing neurotransmitter called acetylcholine. That discovery has prompted recent efforts to try to make up for that loss by administering drugs and nutritional agents that boost the brain's acetylcholine content.

In Parkinson's disease, brain damage mainly targets a particular set of dopamine-producing neurons, shortchanging the body of the dopamine neurotransmitter so essential for controlling muscle movements and balance. One of the most effective drug therapies for patients with Parkinson's is L-Dopa, which helps restore a normal level of that crucial neurotransmitter.

In Part II of *The Brain Wellness Plan,* we describe each neurological disease in relationship to the chemical messengers involved in the brain-immune communication relay systems. Right now, though, we'll simply profile a few of the most important neurotransmitters to emerge among the more than fifty to have been discovered and studied in recent years.

# A Profile of the Brain's Key Players

## • *GABA and Glutamate*

Two of the most abundant neurotransmitters in the central nervous system, glutamate and GABA (gamma-aminobutyric acid) are amino acids that play opposing roles. Because glutamate plays an energizing role while GABA is the calming neurotransmitter, the two are important in maintaining brain health. In addition to playing an energizing role, glutamate acts to stimulate brain cells. However, if your brain should produce excessive amounts of this excitatory neurotransmitter, healthy neurons may be destroyed. GABA, on the other hand, reduces brain cell activity. Depressed levels of this calming neurotransmitter are associated with anxiety and epileptic seizures.

## • *Serotonin*

A neurotransmitter synthesized from the amino acid tryptophan, serotonin is intimately involved in regulating sleep, appetite, sexual behavior, mood, and cardiovascular and immune activity. An imbalance of serotonin may be responsible for depression, autism, obsessive-compulsive disorder, eating disorders, sleep disturbances, and chronic pain syndromes.

## • *Acetylcholine*

Acetylcholine is perhaps the most vital neurotransmitter in regulating memory and cognitive abilities. A depressed level of acetylcholine is the key culprit for the symptoms associated with Alzheimer's disease.

## • *Dopamine*

Dopamine greatly influences your thought processes and motor activity. Low dopamine levels in the brain cause the tremor, impaired motor control, and poor balance that are hallmark symptoms of Parkinson's.

## • Norepinephrine

When you are excited or anxious and feel your heart pounding, it is due to the effects of the brain's norepinephrine messages on your heart. An imbalance of this neurotransmitter may cause impaired physiological responses to stress and other emotional events.

## • Prostaglandins

Originally, these hormone-like molecules were not considered in relation to their impact on the brain. Now research has demonstrated that prostaglandins, which are derived from biological fats (phospholipids), influence the activity of receptors and neurotransmitters.

A key prostaglandin in the brain-immune connection is a substance known as arachidonic acid. Derived from specific types of dietary fats known as omega-6 fatty acids, arachidonic acid is involved in promoting the destructive effects of the neurotransmitter glutamate we described earlier.

## • Nitric Oxide

The newest neurotransmitter to fall under scientific scrutiny, nitric oxide holds exciting promise for maintaining and mending the brain-immune connection. This tiny molecule has an edge over its larger molecular-weight neurotransmitter cousins for two reasons: its small size allows it to diffuse more rapidly through tissues, and it does not require specific cell membrane binding sites for its activity. Instead, nitric oxide rapidly enters cells and works from within cell membranes, which is why we call it a "rapid response neurotransmitter." As you will see throughout *The Brain Wellness Plan,* nitric oxide is deeply involved in learning and memory, and helps coordinate activity between the brain and immune system.

Before proceeding to a more detailed discussion of these and other neurotransmitters, the role they play in causing and treating specific diseases, and complete protocols for aggressively restoring the body's chemical balances, we want to introduce you to your brain's partner in health: your immune system.

## Your Brain's Most Important Partner: The Immune System

The biological complexity of the brain's communication system is matched in intricacy and efficiency by the immune system's complicated communication network. Like the brain, the immune system's different components "speak" to one another—and with the rest of the body—through its chemical messengers, the immunotransmitters.

At its most basic level, the function of the immune system is to protect us from the harmful effects of bacteria, viruses, parasites, and environmental toxins. This enormous task is carried out by various components of the immune system, which must work in close harmony with one another for best results.

The most important of these immune system components are the lymphocytes, or white blood cells, which fight bacteria, fungi, and other foreign bodies. Lymphocytes include both T cells and B cells.

In addition, throughout this book you will read about another important type of white blood cell, the macrophage. Macrophages are the immune system's foot soldiers, capable of engaging in hand-to-hand battle and literally gobbling up invaders to destroy them.

The number of white blood cells called into battle depends, of course, on the severity of the invasion. Your immunotransmitters play a vital role in goading the immune system components into action and in regulating the scope of the battle.

## Cytokines: The Immune System's Messengers

Because the immune system plays such a complex role in defending our bodies, it has developed a highly specialized form of communication to allow its various cellular components to coordinate their ferocious activity. This communication relies on immunotransmitters called cytokines.

Cytokines are to the immune system what neurotransmitters are to the brain. Just as the brain relies on neurotransmitters to exchange information among its own neurons and with the rest of the body, so your immune system's ability to relay messages between its components and throughout the body depends on cytokines.

The three types of cytokines you will read about most in this book will be the interleukins, tumor necrosis factor (TNF), and interferons. All these natural proteins are capable of mounting and amplifying immune responses to a variety of biological challenges.

When your body is threatened by invasion, cytokines signal your immune system to mobilize reserve troops of white blood cells. When the invasion is over, it is up to your cytokines to put out the word to stop mobilizing the troops.

In other words, these immunotransmitters coordinate your white blood cells, boosting their activity at times of infection, injury, or other demands and reining them back in after battle. In this regard, we can think of cytokines as the body's Paul Revere molecules, calling the immune system's troops out as needed.

## The Brain-Immune Connection: A Two-Way Dialogue

In the past, scientists catalogued neurotransmitters as chemical messengers limited only to transmitting information between neurons in the brain. As we explained earlier, however, recent investigations at top research institutions worldwide have dispelled that notion—we now understand that there is a two-way chemical dialogue between the brain and the immune system. Each can influence the other directly.

For example, the neurotransmitters norepinephrine and serotonin have receptors on various components of the immune system and are therefore able to influence immune response in specific ways.

Conversely, in certain areas of the brain, neurons have receptors for cytokines. As you will see in the next chapter, when cytokines are unleashed by the immune system, they can profoundly alter the way important neurotransmitters are released or inhibited.

Another good example of the brain's influence on the immune system is through the cortisol hormone. Cortisol is produced via the hypothalamus. When you suffer stress, your hypothalamus produces a substance called "corticotropin-releasing factor" (CRF), which then stimulates the release of cortisol from your adrenal glands. Cortisol plays such a pivotal role in the brain-immune connection that it has fallen under close scrutiny for its relationship to such diverse disease states as depression, chronic fatigue syndrome, and Alzheimer's.

Why is cortisol so important? The increased level of cortisol triggered by stress—an adaptive response that no doubt evolved to help us survive attacks by predators or enemy tribes—allows your body to muster a coordinated defense to the event. That defense may include heightened awareness, increased heart rate, and increased blood flow to muscles.

Cortisol also has the ability to alter the immune system's production of white blood cells, and to cause them to migrate to particular regions of the body during times of injury, infection, and stress.

## The Brain's Own Immune System

You rarely see the immune system's components in the brain, because an overzealous immune response activated to fight off invading toxins or viruses is all too capable of killing off healthy (and irreplaceable) brain cells in the process.

However, as Drs. Wolfgang J. Streit and Carol A. Kincaid-Colton explain in their November 1995 article in *Scientific American,* scientists are in the throes of discovering mounting evidence for an extensive defense network that functions like the brain's own private immune system.

Studies examining the way certain "microglia" cells respond to antibodies in the brain demonstrate that these normally mild-mannered cells can perform amazing, Superman-like feats.

Within minutes of disturbances in their environment, microglia cells rush to surround damaged neurons and produce some of the same deadly chemicals that immune system cells manufacture to eat up invaders.

As in the immune system, some of those protective chemicals used by the brain's microglia also end up destroying healthy bystander cells in the course of battle. This has aroused new suspicions that overzealous microglia may contribute to certain neurologic disorders.

The possible good news? Finding ways to specifically inhibit microglia activity or block their products might yield new therapies for treating patients with neurological illnesses.

## What's Next?

Now that you understand a bit about your body's essential chemical messengers and how they function to keep you healthy, we will discuss the various roles that neurotransmitters and immunotransmitters play in causing the breakdown of the brain-immune connection that is the hallmark of neurological disease.

# CHAPTER 2

# COMMUNICATION BREAKDOWN

Because every disease we discuss in this book is directly influenced by a brain-immune system communication breakdown, in this chapter we focus on just how disturbances in the brain-immune connection are associated with these diseases.

Like any partnership, the brain-immune relationship can become strained and damaging to both parties if communication breaks down. Several important factors appear to be responsible for causing communication to falter between these systems— factors based on the unique characteristics of the two systems involved.

The brain, for instance, is a very fatty substance. Approximately 25 percent of the dry weight of the brain is composed of lipids (fats). These lipids serve many important roles, which include insulating nerve fibers and acting as the building blocks of cell membranes surrounding neurons.

As essential as these brain cell lipids may be to your brain's health, however, the brain's fatty content has a downside as well: it makes the brain an easy target for immune-initiated injury through free radical attack.

Other natural agents called upon by the immune system in defending the body against diseases, infections, toxins, and other stresses may also serve as catalysts for devastating neurological illnesses. These include nitric oxide, one of the newest neuro-transmitters to demand the scientific spotlight; cytokines, the immune system's most important immunotransmitters; and cortisol, the hormone which plays such a principal role in mediating the body's response to stress.

Contemporary scientific studies in neurology and immunology have demonstrated that the body's own immune system has the ability to damage healthy brain cells. As you will discover in *The Brain Wellness Plan,* the failure of your own body's natural ability to protect itself against an inappropriate immune response may lead to neurological illnesses such as Parkinson's, Alzheimer's, and Lou Gehrig's disease.

## The Body's Terrorists: Rampaging Free Radicals

When the body fights off an infection, the immune system's cytokines go to work, sending messages to the brain that cause more white blood cells to mobilize. The more white blood cells your body activates, the more free radicals they produce.

These free radicals are among your immune system's most powerful weapons. Naturally produced by the body as a response to aging and during times of disease, injury, and emotional stress, free radicals are chemicals with a single electron molecule, whose mission it is to find another electron free for pairing. That process of electron looting is known as "oxidation," and it's the same process that rusts metal and spoils butter.

Various components of the immune system rely on free radicals to neutralize threatening invaders. Free radicals are like pellets of poison pinging about in the body, damaging whatever they hit. These free radicals go to work to destroy invaders by interfering with their cellular machinery, literally dissolving or breaking down the genetic material of bacteria, toxins, and viruses.

When all is going well, the immune system is capable of identifying foreign invaders such as viruses and bacteria by accurately "reading" molecular codes found on cell surfaces. These molecular codes are like the flags of different armies, and the immune system will not attack a cell if it sees a flag belonging to the body's own host army.

Once the immune system has produced antibodies to a certain antigen, or invader, it even develops a "memory" of sorts, so that it can readily respond with the same fighter cells the next time that invader appears.

If functioning properly, then, our immune components do not turn against our own body's cells. Unfortunately, free radicals can interfere with the biological components of our own healthy cells just as they destroy invaders, literally dismantling the body's essential cellular proteins, fatty cell membranes, and DNA. And too often, the cells destroyed by free radicals are in the brain, because the high fat content of the brain's neurons make them particularly vulnerable to free radical attack.

Why is fat so attractive to free radicals? Because fat, by its very chemical makeup—it contains carbon, oxygen, and hydrogen molecules—can readily give up an electron to a free radical in search of a partner. And then that fat molecule, in turn, becomes a free radical, perpetuating the cycle of free radical destruction.

This process is called "lipid peroxidation," which means that the fat literally becomes oxidized and goes from being a stable molecule to an unstable molecule. We see it as a biological uprising, where just one free radical has the ability to attract others to its revolutionary cause and produce instability in the biological government.

The most important natural defenses we have against free radical damage are our body's natural "antioxidants," a broad range of chemical substances that all have one thing in common: they ward off free radical damage to cells because they can safely donate electrons. Pairing those antioxidant electrons with free radicals effectively stops free radicals in their tracks—often in time to prevent damage to healthy cells.

The brain has a highly developed antioxidant security system designed to protect itself against free radical attack. This antioxidant system involves two critical enzymes, superoxide dismutase and glutathione, which you will hear more about later. These two substances are the front line body guards capable of protecting the delicate machinery of neurons from the harmful effects of free radicals.

Unfortunately, in many neurological diseases—including Parkinson's, Alzheimer's, ALS, and multiple sclerosis—the brain's specialized antioxidant mechanisms fail. As you will see in Part II, the cause of this failure might be genetic, environmental, or even dietary, but the consequences are the same: unchecked free radical activity on the brain's cellular machinery.

This free radical attack hones in on the fat-heavy membranes of the brain's neurons. When a neuron membrane undergoes lipid peroxidation, the fats acquire more oxygen and become rancid (peroxidized). This causes a chain reaction, causing those neurons to break down and destroy surrounding healthy brain cells in turn.

Lipid peroxidation appears to be the final common pathway for many neurological illnesses. Specific disease symptoms depend on which area of the brain is under attack.

In Alzheimer's, for instance, the cell membranes of the hippocampus, the brain's memory region, are the ones to fall prey to free radical attack. In Parkinson's disease, on the other hand, the area of the brain to suffer the most damage is the "substantia nigra," which produces dopamine, the neurotransmitter responsible for muscle movement and coordination.

In addition, certain investigators have shown that free radical attack on one of the fatty substances found in brain cells—arachidonic acid—can literally accelerate the free radical injury to brain cells.

Arachidonic acid is normally kept under a tight lock and key by neurons. However, during excessive immune system activity and free radical production, arachidonic acid is released and stimulates a series of injurious steps to brain cells. The most potentially damaging effect of arachidonic acid is its ability to create an extensive amount of glutamate, the excitatory neurotransmitter that researchers have linked to ALS and Parkinson's disease.

## The Role of Nitric Oxide in Producing the Most Toxic Free Radical Offender of All

In the last chapter, you read about the value of nitric oxide as a neurotransmitter. Unfortunately, the excessive production of nitric oxide can also be blamed for throwing the brain-immune connection off kilter and causing some of the brain's worst free radical damage.

When the immune system's cytokines activate the macrophages—those important white blood cells capable of gobbling up invading viruses and bacteria—the macrophages produce large amounts of nitric oxide in the course of battle.

Over the past decade, scientists have shown that the production of nitric oxide through the combination of immune and nervous system activity—activity often sparked by an infection, exposure to a toxin, or as part of the aging process—plays a key role in the development of neurological diseases.

The real trouble starts when nitric oxide, through various chemical reactions, produces peroxynitrite, a biologically essential oxidant with the dubious distinction of being the most toxic free radical to the body—and especially to the brain.

For instance, recent studies of human plasma exposed to peroxynitrite show that this free radical terrorist is capable of damaging plasma proteins and depleting such crucial antioxidants as vitamin C, uric acid, coenzyme Q10, and glutathione. Peroxynitrite also has the potential to step up the production of toxic lipid peroxides which further damage cell membranes.

You will read more about peroxynitrite in the next chapter and in our chapter on Parkinson's disease. There, we discuss new scientific evidence supporting the idea that inhibiting nitric oxide synthesis may prevent the loss of dopamine-producing neurons because it slows down peroxynitrite production.

## How Cytokines Play a Role in Disease

Cytokines—the immune system's own chemical messengers crafted to deliver warnings to speed up or slow down the immune system's responses—may also play a complex role in causing or promoting neurological illness.

How do they do this? Researchers have discovered that certain cytokines are specifically "offensive" because they ratchet up immune system activity.

In recent years, investigators have identified a large number of cytokines as the cause of quite a few—and sometimes detrimental—effects on brain function. For example, certain cytokines are capable of producing fatigue, slowed thinking, and other depressive symptoms. The gamma interferon cytokine directly inhibits the brain's ability to synthesize serotonin, and low levels of serotonin can cause depression. This may explain why patients with viral illnesses or diseases such as multiple sclerosis experience much higher rates of depression, as low serotonin levels are directly linked to depressive states.

In addition, we now have evidence that the cytokine interleukin-1 promotes sleep and reduces appetite. In patients with Alzheimer's disease, scientists have demonstrated that interleukin-6 is partially responsible for the manufacture of beta amyloid, one of the substances that kills off brain cells and destroys memory.

## Cortisol: Too Much of a Good Thing Causes Problems

As you learned in the last chapter, cortisol is the hormone that allows your body to coordinate a response to stress. Typically, when that stress abates, your sensory organs send a message to your brain that it's okay to shut down cortisol production for the time being. However, under some circumstances, the cortisol response ends up perpetuating itself, resulting in a variety of pathological changes in the brain and immune system.

What happens when your body's cells are continually exposed to cortisol? Studies reveal that continued exposure to excessive cortisol may damage specific brain regions involved in mood and memory. In addition, your body's immune mechanisms may automatically shut down when too much cortisol is present.

## Preprogrammed Cell Death

In order for the body to stay healthy, millions of our cells sacrifice themselves every minute as part of the brain's natural, ongoing housekeeping process to keep things in order.

Scientists have now discovered that certain groups of brain cells are destined for a preprogrammed cell death. This mysterious form of cell suicide is called "apoptosis," from the Greek for "a flower losing its petals."

A number of brain disorders, including Alzheimer's, Parkinson's, and amyotrophic lateral sclerosis, may result when apoptosis spins out of control and leads to abnormal cell suicide. Investigators believe apoptosis is mediated by specific immune system cytokines known as interleukins. If so, learning to inhibit inappropriate apoptosis with neuroimmunomodulating nutritional substances, hormones, and drugs will no doubt contribute to new therapies for neurological illnesses in the future.

## What's Next: Basic Nutritional Guidelines

Now that you know just how important it is to maintain a healthy brain-immune connection, you're probably wondering how to get started on just the right foods and supplements for optimum health.

In the next chapter, we discuss your body's gastrointestinal tract in relation to its brain-supporting role, and present a basic nutritional guideline for brain wellness that every healthy individual should incorporate into a daily nutritional plan.

# FOOD FOR THOUGHT

In this chapter, we focus on the first part of our two-step Brain Wellness Plan, the nutritional guidelines any healthy individual must follow to support optimum overall health. First, however, we will take a quick look at the body's digestive tract.

Wait: if this is a book about the brain, why are we bothering to include information on your digestive tract?

Simple. The gastrointestinal (GI) tract carries out three important roles in maintaining an optimum brain-immune connection. First of all, the brain absolutely depends on the GI tract's ability to assimilate and deliver nutrients which act as essential building blocks for neurotransmitters. Secondly, the brain requires the GI tract to remove toxins which have the potential to adversely affect brain-immune function. And, finally, optimum brain health rests on the GI tract's ability to properly regulate immune system activity.

## Why is a Healthy Gastrointestinal Tract so Important for the Brain?

• *The Brain is a Hungry Organ.*

The idea that your brain's metabolism is highly dependent on your body's overall nutritional status becomes evident if you think about your brain's neurons—like all cells in your body—as tiny factories. Each neuron shoulders the responsibility for producing its own energy and requires certain nutrients to fuel its manufacturing processes.

Every cell is made up of carbohydrate, protein, and fat molecules, and most of a cell's metabolism is carried out within its mitochondria. These tiny organelles are often referred to by biologists as "the powerhouses of the cell" because mitochondria are so important to oxidative phosphorylation—the chemical production of energy and a fundamental process to all living creatures that need oxygen.

Because of their complex communication duties, neurons consume an average of five times more glucose than other cells in the body. For that kind of fuel, the brain must depend on the digestive tract's efficient intestinal digestion and absorption of food.

In recent years, many in the scientific community have devoted their research to documenting the relationship between nutrients and brain cell function. The brain is dependent on adequate gastrointestinal function for delivering the essential nutrients it cannot make on its own. Otherwise, the brain will not be able to keep its biological machinery running.

In addition to providing the essential compounds for cellular energy production, the GI tract must also deliver the ingredients for other critical brain constituents. These include essential fatty acids, or phospholipids, which act as building blocks for cell membranes, hormones, and certain neurotransmitters.

The GI tract also carries B vitamins to the brain. B vitamins are indispensable in synthesizing neurotransmitters and in forming myelin, the insulating substance that sheaths connections between neurons and makes it possible for them to transmit messages effectively.

### • The Brain Relies on the GI Tract to Help Clean House

Your gastrointestinal tract always has different types of resident bacteria—some useful to our digestive processes, some harmful. A second, and equally essential, role the GI tract plays in brain function therefore involves maintaining a healthy ecological balance between beneficial and harmful bacteria. The GI tract's natural detoxification processes allow most harmful toxins to exit the body via the liver.

If the GI tract should fail to keep up with its housekeeping chores, a variety of toxins produced by certain strains of bacteria may have detrimental consequences on brain metabolism. These toxins can eventually produce a variety of neurological and psychiatric symptoms, ranging from seizures to behavioral disturbances.

Of all the toxins to reach the brain as a result of impaired GI function, ammonia is the best documented. Normally produced in the GI tract by bacteria as a result of protein digestion, ammonia is cleaned out of healthy bodies through the liver, which serves as the body's major detoxification center.

In patients with liver disease, high levels of ammonia have been linked to deleterious effects on brain function. In fact, patients with elevated ammonia levels due to an impaired GI tract may suffer from personality changes, agitation, hyperactivity, and seizures.

Recently, scientists have also uncovered links between bacterially derived toxins in the GI tract and neurological diseases such as schizophrenia and autism. In schizophrenia, some researchers have speculated that specific substances manufactured by anaerobic bacteria in the GI tract interfere with synaptophysin, an important brain protein required for the release of certain neurotransmitters.

And in patients with autism, specific organic acids released by different strains of bacteria appear to interfere with the brain's ability to properly metabolize glucose.

## The Gut–Immune System Connection

Rather than think of the immune system as outside and separate from the gut, think of your GI tract as part of your immune system in the way it protects the body from disease.

Groups of nerve fibers line the intestinal wall from the esophagus to the rectum. More than half of your immune system occupies the space surrounding the gastrointestinal tract, making the GI tract the largest organ in the body capable of producing important immune system components such as white blood cells and cytokines.

Since most microorganisms that threaten the body enter through the mouth and nose, the GI tract also acts as a main line of immune defense, preventing microscopic invaders and other materials contained in the intestinal tract from passing into the body's internal environment.

Its exposure to many antigens causes the GI tract's immune response to be activated regularly. If the immune response that takes place in the GI tract were separate from the rest of the immune system, this would pose no problem. The gut could simply respond to an invader without the dramatic domino effect of gearing up an entire systemic immune response with all of those potential consequences, like inflammation.

In essence, then, your GI tract acts as a neuroimmunomodulating organ by supporting a healthy immune system response to infections, toxins, and other stresses. However, if the GI tract is not healthy, the consequences may be devastating, in that your entire immune system kicks into gear and affects the rest of your body systems. Many brain-immune disorders are directly or indirectly related to dysfunctions in the GI tract—largely because your gut's failure to do its job of utilizing nutrients and cleansing the body of harmful substances can result in inappropriate immune system activation.

## How Does the GI Tract Communicate?

Just as the brain and immune system communicate through chemical messengers, your GI tract relies on specific substances called peptides to relay information. These are long sequences of amino acids that we find widely distributed in the brain and gastrointestinal tract. Peptides can be readily absorbed from the gastrointestinal tract, entering the bloodstream and eventually reaching the brain.

Once they have successfully completed their winding journey into the brain, peptides regulate the synthesis of new neurotransmitters, influencing the metabolism of brain cells.

We now believe that peptides are able to modulate our pain, memory, learning, and behavior—which is why peptide function is currently the subject of top-funded clinical and basic science research investigations into neurological disorders.

## Food for Thought: From Theory to Practice

*The Brain Wellness Plan* is a two-step process that focuses on general dietary guidelines. We developed these guidelines to help ensure that you can adequately incorporate and assimilate (1) the nutrients any healthy individual should include in a diet designed to support optimum health and (2) specific brain-supporting substances we recommend for individuals eager to prevent neurological illnesses by boosting the brain-immune connection. We call these therapeutic substances "neuroimmunomodulators."

We will discuss specific neuroimmunomodulators, or Step 2 of *The Brain Wellness Plan,* in the next chapter. They will appear again in relation to specific diseases in Part II of this book.

For now, however, we will focus only on practical, general nutritional guidelines every person should follow as the first step toward maintaining lifelong optimum brain function.

## A Nutrition Primer for Brain-Immune Health: Basic Guidelines for the Healthy Individual

Ask your physician, best friends, and family members to describe the perfect diet, and you're likely to get as many different descriptions of an "ideal" regimen as the number of people you ask. This shouldn't be surprising, since even many physicians and clinical nutritionists hotly disagree about the "perfect" foods and nutritional supplements.

What most professionals in nutritional science *will* unite to tell you, however, is that the Recommended Daily Allowances (RDAs) touted for so long by the government as the gold standard of nutrition are really nothing more than a shadowy list of minimum requirements.

The RDA is a blueprint for preventing vitamin deficiencies, but shortchanges you when it comes to listing optimum doses of all the nutrients necessary for healthy brain and immune system function. And when it comes to preventing and treating diseases of any kind, the RDAs fail utterly.

At the end of this chapter, you will find a summary chart that serves as a quick source and dosage guide for optimal brain-immune nutrients. You should address specific recommendations with your health care practitioner.

## Getting Started on the Road to Health

- Avoid current fad diets and focus on your individual health profile—seek the guidance of a clinical nutritionist.
- Eat a variety of foods, with emphasis on dark-colored fruits and vegetables such as blueberries, cantaloupe, broccoli, kale, tomatoes, and sweet potatoes.
- Eat whole, unrefined, nutrient-dense carbohydrates such as whole grain bread, cereals, pasta, brown rice, oats, barley, etc.
- Eat organic vegetables, meats, or poultry to avoid exposure to excessive hormones and pesticides.
- Limit your fat intake to a maximum of 25 percent of your total daily calories.
  - Limit saturated fats, such as butter and fats found in milk and meat, to no more than 5 percent of your fat intake.
  - Emphasize monounsaturated fats (such as olive oil) and fats high in omega-3 fatty acids (flaxseed oil, fish oils) to constitute the remaining 20 percent of your fat intake.
- Limit red meats to no more than 4 ounces two times per week.
- Emphasize fish, fowl, and low-fat yogurt as protein sources.
- Explore vegetarian sources of protein, including tofu, tempeh, wheat gluten, and grain and bean dishes.

- Limit cholesterol to less than 300 mg daily.
- Avoid sugar and sweets.
- Do not be fooled by the new "low-fat" desserts, as they are usually loaded with sugar.
- Avoid packaged, processed foods that may contain undesirable nutritional constituents such as hydrogenated fats, preservatives, or high amounts of saturated fat or sugar.

## How Can You Help Your GI Tract Absorb Brain Nutrients?

As we learned earlier in this chapter, your GI tract plays an indispensable part in absorbing and delivering essential nutrients to the brain. Unfortunately, all it takes is a brief look at the shelves of your local pharmacy to know that most people are not digesting nutrients very well: those stomach remedies, antacids, laxatives, and digestive aids add up to a billion-dollar industry.

In other words, you aren't "what you eat," as perhaps your mother once cautioned you. More accurately, you are "what you use," or what you can digest and absorb.

As you now know, the health of your GI tract affects the digestion, absorption, and function of many nutritional substances. Additionally, your GI tract is the first line of defense against disease-causing bacteria and viruses. Therefore, your GI tract is an integral aspect of your immune defense in maintaining wellness. That's why good digestion is as crucial to your health as optimum nutrition.

Enhancing your GI tract's ability to perform its brain-supporting duties requires a combination of substances, including glutamine, dietary fiber, friendly bacteria, chlorophyll, and nucleotides. While these nutrients may not directly affect brain health, they do support the GI tract functions so essential to brain wellness.

### •Glutamine

An important amino acid, glutamine is the major source of energy for cells in the GI tract and important to protein synthesis.

Glutamine helps preserve the integrity of the GI tract by maintaining its mucosal barrier lining and thus keeping toxins out of the bloodstream and away from the brain.

Glutamine is also the primary respiratory fuel for stimulated macrophages and lymphocytes. Finally, it has been identified as a critical nutrient for maintaining the immune system and for preventing bacteria from leaving the gut following injury or other trauma.

While you can find glutamine in protein-containing foods, we recommend supplements of this vital gut-supporting nutrient.

> **RECOMMENDED DOSE FOR HEALTHY INDIVIDUALS:** 1000 mg daily. Take on an empty stomach to maximize absorption.

## • Indigestible Fiber

Indigestible fiber helps you eliminate wastes and harmful bacterial toxins from the GI tract. Also, increased intake of these dietary fibers helps stimulate the growth of beneficial bacteria and repair colon cells. The dietary guidelines we recommend here will be useful in providing valuable fibers to the diet.

Using special indigestible fibers such as fructosoligosaccarides (FOS) can provide an important medium in the large intestine for feeding beneficial bacteria. You can purchase FOS by itself or combined with friendly bacteria.

> **RECOMMENDED DOSE FOR HEALTHY INDIVIDUALS:** 4 g of FOS daily in addition to dietary fiber from meals. May be taken in divided doses between meals.

## • Friendly Bacteria

The gut's integrity is also maintained by a healthy balance of "friendly" microorganisms such as those found in the lactobacillus and bifido bacteria families. Maintaining high levels of these friendly bacteria in the intestinal tract is critical for detoxification and health. By producing acids and natural antibiotics, warding off pathogens such as viruses and molds, and assisting your GI tract in proper bowel function, these friendly bacteria play important roles in keeping your entire system healthy.

> **RECOMMENDED DOSE FOR HEALTHY INDIVIDUALS:** Look for supplements containing billions of both lactobacillus and bifido strains of the beneficial bacteria. We recommend following the dosages typically found in the product's "suggested use" section. It is best to take these products between meals.

## • Chlorophyll

Products such as wheat, barley, and oat grass powders are rich in chlorophyll—a substance known for its power to remove toxins from your intestinal tract.

> **RECOMMENDED DOSE FOR HEALTHY INDIVIDUALS:** We suggest supplementing your diet with a high-chlorophyll drink such as wheat grass juice or barley grass juice once or twice daily, between meals. These are also available in tablets.

## • Nucleotides

Nucleotides are the structural units of nucleic acids, and play a major role in almost every one of your body's biochemical processes.

You are probably most familiar with nucleotides as the building blocks of our genetic material: DNA (deoxyribonucleic acid) and RNA (ribonucleic acid). Chemically, nucleotides are known as cytidine, adenosine, guanine, inosine, and uridine.

Essentially, a healthy brain–gut–immune system feedback loop depends on the efficient function of your body's nucleotides, as these acids modify the type and growth of intestinal bacteria. Specifically, nucleotides enhance the growth of "friendly" bacteria, such as lactobacilli and bifido, in the gastrointestinal tract, and suppress the proliferation of the "bad" bacteria that can provoke an immune system response.

Investigators have demonstrated that nucleotides are important for maintaining cellular immune response, and their deficiency may impair that. Today's clinical studies with human subjects confirm the benefits of dietary nucleotides, which are now used to supplement hospital feedings and infant formulas. All foods with protein contain nucleotides, and infants receive them naturally through breast milk.

RECOMMENDED DOSE FOR HEALTHY INDIVIDUALS: To benefit most from nucleotides—especially when your immune system is challenged during infections—we recommend supplementing your diet with nucleotides in the 1–2 g range. Nucleotides should be taken between meals for the most efficient absorption.

## Basic Brain Nutrients

### • Multivitamins

The "multi" is the basis for any supplement program and represents an overall "insurance" supplement to the diet by providing a wide array of essential nutrients. You'll find a variety of multis on the market. Basically, multivitamins come in one-, two-, or three-a-day formulas and in tablet or capsule form. Essentially, all cover the same spectrum of nutrients.

RECOMMENDED DOSE FOR HEALTHY INDIVIDUALS: Our preference is for the two- or three-a-day formula multivitamins. Taken in smaller amounts throughout the day, the nutrients are better absorbed and utilized than if taken all at once.

### • Antioxidants

A full spectrum of antioxidants—including carotenoids, vitamin E, vitamin C, polyphenols, lipoic acid, n-acetyl-cysteine, tocotrienols, and coenzyme Q10—is your best support against free radical damage to the body. We will discuss specific neuroimmunomodulating antioxidants in greater detail in the next chapter.

*RECOMMENDED DOSE FOR HEALTHY INDIVIDUALS:* We recommend adding any one of the general antioxidant supplements on the market to the general multiple vitamin, since the antioxidant supplement contains higher quantities and a more complete array of this important class of nutrients.

## • Calcium-Magnesium Supplement

While these minerals have been emphasized for healthy bones and marketed to women, calcium and magnesium also play important roles in maintaining brain wellness. Magnesium plays a pivotal role in brain cell energy production by activating crucial enzymes involved in the manufacture of ATP, the energy currency of cells. Magnesium is also an important ingredient for the enzymes essential in producing important neurotransmitters such as serotonin.

In addition, magnesium stabilizes cell membranes and protects them against the harmful effects of excitatory neurotransmitters such as glutamate, and has been documented for its beneficial effects in preventing migraine headaches. Calcium, meanwhile, is a critical mineral for boosting the potential of nerve and muscle cells to communicate through electrical impulses.

*RECOMMENDED DOSE FOR HEALTHY INDIVIDUALS:* Because calcium and magnesium are too large to be contained in sufficient quantities in the general multivitamin supplements on the market, we recommend taking 1000 mg of calcium and 500 mg of magnesium daily. Each of these minerals is available individually or may be purchased together in a single formulation. For your convenience, you may wish to purchase the combination calcium-magnesium products.

## • The B Vitamins: More than Just Deficiency Fighters

The entire group of B vitamins is involved in maintaining a healthy brain-immune connection. The major B vitamins include thiamine (B1), riboflavin (B2), niacin (B3), pyridoxine (B6), cobalamin (B12), folic acid, pantothenic acid, biotin, choline, and inositol.

The B vitamins work in chorus to promote brain and immune system health by protecting nerve tissue against oxidation, enhancing memory, and insulating nerve cells. Your body also requires B vitamins for producing many neurotransmitters. Choline and phosphatidylcholine, for example, are necessary for the brain's manufacture of acetylcholine, the memory neurotransmitter that runs short in Alzheimer's disease and other disorders.

Scientists have long recognized the symptoms of B vitamin deficiency. Some of those include many of the same symptoms associated with Alzheimer's and other dementias, such as memory loss, emotional instability, and reduced attention span.

For instance, recent studies have shown that the important neurotransmitters GABA and serotonin require adequate levels of vitamin B6 to be properly synthesized by the brain's neurons.

The brain requires adequate thiamine from the diet to effectively use carbohydrates for energy production. In addition, dietary B12 and folic acid are both necessary to form myelin, the insulating substance that sheathes neurons and makes it possible for neurons to transmit messages.

Links between nutritional disorders and neurological clinical symptoms have also been well documented. A severe thiamine deficiency can result in hallucinations and memory disturbances, while a shortage of vitamin B6 leads to irritability, depression, and seizures. A vitamin B12 deficiency can result in memory disturbances and impaired sensations.

We cannot overemphasize the importance of adequate B vitamin intake for a healthy nervous system and proper brain function. The best dietary sources include whole grain breads, cereals, pastas, and meat. We also suggest adding a complete B vitamin supplement to the diet instead of incorporating large doses of individual B vitamins.

**RECOMMENDED DOSE FOR HEALTHY INDIVIDUALS:** A daily supplement that provides 50 mg each of the entire family of B vitamins.

### • Copper, Zinc, Manganese, and Selenium: Essential Micronutrients to Incorporate Into Your Diet

Four of the most important micronutrients that healthy individuals should consider adding as daily supplements are copper, zinc, manganese, and selenium.

The distribution of copper in the brain corresponds directly to the distribution of the neurons that synthesize dopamine and norepinephrine, for example. This makes sense, since the enzyme that serves as an essential ingredient for synthesizing those neurotransmitters is copper-dependent.

Zinc, an essential trace mineral found in protein-rich foods such as meat and whole grains, has a number of important effects on the brain. Among them are zinc's influence on neurotransmitter production and enzyme functioning. It is interesting to note that the brain's highest concentration of zinc is located in the hippocampus, the brain's memory center.

If children suffer a zinc deficiency, they may experience appetite disturbances and growth retardation. Zinc also plays a leading role in preventing brain damage in children exposed to lead at an early age.

A combination of zinc, copper, and manganese is essential in inducing the important cellular antioxidant, superoxidase dismutase (SOD). Like glutathione, SOD is responsible for protecting cells from free radical damage. It is important to note, however, that individuals with Parkinson's disease should avoid taking manganese supplements at all; we discuss this further in our chapter on that illness.

Finally, selenium has the ability to increase the production of glutathione, a key intracellular antioxidant enzyme system responsible for protecting all of the body's cells from free radical damage and detoxifying noxious agents from the body.

**RECOMMENDED DOSES FOR HEALTHY INDIVIDUALS:** Because these micronutrients are so essential to your health, we recommend adding supplements of each to your daily diet. Look for fully reacted mineral chelates for each of the minerals recommended below.

| | |
|---|---|
| Copper | 2 mg |
| Zinc | 30 mg (adults); 15 mg (children 6–12) |

Selenium     200 mcg (Do not exceed this amount.)
Manganese    2 mg (except for those with Parkinson's
             disease)

Each of these nutrients should be taken daily with a meal.

This is just a partial list of the many nutrients we now know are essential to maintaining an optimum brain-immune connection. We have outlined recommended food sources and dosages of all these nutrients in Table 1.

## What's Next: Using Neuroimmunomodulators to Mend the Brain-Immune Connection

As you have seen, research conducted at major medical centers and universities around the world has shown that disturbances in the balance of our body's fatty acids and destruction of healthy brain cells by free radicals lie at the heart of disease.

Combining expert knowledge of these culprits with our new-found understanding of the power of nutrients to maintain and restore the brain-immune connection, we now turn our attention to the second step of our Brain Wellness Plan. This step relies on neuroimmunomodulators.

Informed clinicians from around the world are now recommending these nutrients as a means of preventing neurological illness, and are incorporating them into disease therapies designed to treat neurological illnesses.

When combined with advanced medical interventions, these nutritional and hormonal substances have the potential to restore the brain-immune connection. What's more, many are readily available in your local health food store or nutritionally oriented pharmacy.

TABLE  **1**

## GENERAL SUPPLEMENT HEALTH PROTOCOL: A SUMMARY

| Nutrient* | Recommended Daily Dose |
|---|---|
| Multiple vitamin-mineral | Follow label directions. |
| Chelated calcium | 1000 mg, with a meal |
| Chelated magnesium | 500 mg, with a meal |
| Advanced antioxidant formula | Look for an advanced formula and follow label instructions. |

SOD Inducers
(May be obtained individually or found in a single product. Those with Parkinson's should avoid manganese.)

| Copper | 1 mg, with a meal |
|---|---|
| Zinc | 10 mg, with a meal |
| Manganese | 4 mg, with a meal |
| Selenium | 200 mcg, with a meal (Do not exceed this amount.) |

*With regard to all the minerals listed above, look for fully reacted mineral chelates for maximum absorption and utilization.

## GENERAL GUT HEALTH PROTOCOL: A SUMMARY

| Nutrient | Recommended Daily Dose |
|---|---|
| Glutamine | 1000 mg, away from food |
| Multiple strain friendly bacteria | Follow label directions |
| FOS | 4 grams as directed on label |
| Nucleotides | 1–2 grams, away from food |
| Barley grass/wheat grass | 1–2 servings as directed |

# CHAPTER 4

# THE BRAIN
# WELLNESS PLAN

The revolution in neuroimmunomodulation combines studies from nutrition, neurology, and immunology to bring us incredible insights into just how food and supplements can positively influence brain and immune system health.

In this book, we have collected the latest research in designing a basic "Brain Wellness Plan" that serves as a preventive measure for healthy individuals.

Medical science has also demonstrated that certain neuroimmunomodulating agents are also therapeutic in treating neurological diseases. In the next section of the book, we will begin describing those agents disease-by-disease, devoting a chapter to each of the most common neurological ilnesses affecting Americans today.

For now, we will begin by describing the three foundations for brain health. These include (1) the essential fatty acids for the brain and their supporting agents; (2) the body's detoxifying mechanisms, which include a new and powerful generation of antioxidants capable of crossing the blood-brain barrier and s-adenosyl methionine (SAM), a naturally occurring, high-energy body detoxifier; and (3) the DHEA hormone.

## The First Foundation for Brain Health: Fatty Acids

Fatty acids play a key role in brain health and disease because they are so adundant in nervous tissue, including the brain's gray matter and white matter, the myelin sheaths.

Also part of phospholipids, fatty acids serve as building blocks for the cell membranes of neurons and serve as a major constituent of hormones. They are involved in both energy production for cells and neurotransmitter function.

Because fatty acids are the primary components of neuron cell membranes, maintaining them is the first foundation for brain health. The essential phospholipids help ensure the structural foundation of brain cells by forming a protective barrier, preserving the cell's internal milieu and guarding against the potentially harmful effects of toxins.

The composition of the fatty acids that make up brain cell membranes determines the way neurotransmitters bind to membrane receptors. Fatty acids also regulate the opening and closing of channels in and out of brain cells, thus affecting the flow of vital nutrients.

You are at the helm when it comes to determining which fatty acids make up your brain cell membranes, as these fatty acids are largely determined by the fats you consume. In other words, the fatty acids in your diet impact the way neuron membranes function. Even slight alterations in your fatty acid intake may affect the structural integrity of membranes and the way your membrane receptors receive neurotransmitters.

How, then, can you ensure that the fatty acids and phosopholipids in your brain cell membranes are the right ones? First of all, it's important to know that the phosopholipids derived from saturated fat have a considerably different effect on brain membrane function than the phosopholipids derived from unsaturated fatty acids. Basically, the higher the degree of unsaturated fatty acids in your brain cells, the more fluid their membranes will be, allowing for more efficient transport of substances in and out of cells and better communication between neurons.

The essential fatty acids, which are primarily unsaturated fatty acids, are divided into two broad categories, the omega-6 and omega-3 fatty acids.

### •Omega-6 Fatty Acids

Omega-6 fats, which we consume mostly from corn oil and certain vegetable oils, are processed by certain enzymes in the body to make prostaglandins, the hormone-like substances that help regulate immune function.

Prostaglandins derived from omega-6 fats have the potential to be converted to either pro-inflammatory or anti-inflammatory substances, which means they can either cause the immune system response to increase or decrease, respectively.

For example, arachidonic acid, which we discussed earlier, is a pro-inflammatory acid derived from the omega-6 fatty acids. Arachidonic acid plays a primary role in brain injury due to aging, stroke, epilepsy, and various other neurodegenerative diseases. This is because arachidonic acid promotes free radical activity in the body and on brain cells in particular. This acid also enhances the harmful effects of glutamate, the excitatory neurotransmitter linked to Alzheimer's, Parkinson's, and certain forms of epilepsy.

Eating omega-6 fatty acids does not necessarily mean that your body will convert them to arachidonic acid. This is because it takes a special enzyme, known as delta-5 desaturase, to determine whether omega-6 fatty acids will ultimately break down to arachidonic acid. While there is no need to eliminate corn and vegetable oils from the diet completely, we do encourage all of our *Brain Wellness Plan* readers to consider limiting their intake of omega-6 fatty acids for some of the better choices we discuss below.

Obviously, then, controlling the delta-5 desaturase enzyme in the diet is one critical factor in determining the effect of dietary fatty acids on brain function. So what controls this enzyme?

Happily, the answer is at hand in your grocery store and through supplements: the omega-3 fatty acids.

### • Omega-3 Fatty Acids

Readily available in fish and flaxseed oil, omega-3 fatty acids such as EPA (eicosapentaneoic acid) and DHA (docosahexanoic acid) have the potential to support brain and immune function. EPA and DHA are natural anti-inflammatory substances which are able to reduce the potentially harmful effects of arachidonic acid through their ability to inhibit the delta-5 desaturase enzyme.

Throughout this book, you will find disease-specific evidence of the healing powers of the omega-3 fatty acids, especially DHA—knowledge we have gleaned from scientific studies conducted in medical centers and research institutes around the world.

Good sources of omega-3 fats include fatty fish (salmon, tuna, mackerel, and herring), and omega-3 supplements such as flaxseed oil, MaxEPA™ fish oil products, and Neuromins™, a trademarked vegetarian source of pure DHA material. Neuromins™ is a product of Martek Biosciences Corporation and obtained from algae rather than fish; look for this trademarked raw material on the label of your favorite DHA supplement manufacturer.

Of all the omega-3 fatty acids, probably the one you will read about most in this book is DHA. DHA is the primary structural fatty acid in the gray matter of the brain and promotes communication between brain cells by allowing synapses to remain soft and functional.

Recent studies have demonstrated that the lower concentration of omega-3 fatty acids found in infant formulas versus breast milk is linked to lower intelligence in children who consumed those formulas. In 1993, both the Food and Agricultural Organization and the World Health Organization acknowledged DHA's importance in brain development. As a result of recent important research, DHA is now being added to infant formulas.

A naturally anti-inflammatory agent, DHA protects cell membranes against oxidative damage and is being actively examined for its potential in treating clinical conditions ranging from Alzheimer's disease to multiple sclerosis and attention deficit disorder (ADD).

Another naturally occurring fatty acid in the brain and in all cell membranes, PS (phosphatidylserine), has proven to be a safe, potentially effective therapeutic agent in treating memory deficit disorders such as Alzheimer's.

PS enhances enzymes involved in monitoring neurotransmitter production and release. It also increases the brain's energy efficiency because it enhances the brain's ability to metabolize glucose.

Furthermore, PS and DHA can modulate the fluidity of cell membranes—an essential feature if cells are going to "speak" to one another by sending chemical messengers back and forth. PS also increases communication between cells by increasing the number of membrane receptor sites for receiving messages.

As you will see in later chapters, scientific studies have demonstrated that PS supplements can increase the output of acetylcholine, the neurotransmitter so important to memory, and so may enhance the quality of life among Alzheimer's patients. This remarkable substance also has the potential to stimulate the brain to produce dopamine.

Clinical trials with elderly patients suffering memory deficit disorders have shown that adding PS to the daily diet improved the ability of these patients to think and decreased behavioral disturbances. In other studies, PS also improved the performance of patients with age-associated memory impairment, a disorder affecting millions of American each year.

Because PS is such an important neuroimmunomodulator, you will find its therapeutic use—and studies supporting that use—related to a number of disorders described throughout this book.

*RECOMMENDED DOSE FOR HEALTHY INDIVIDUALS:* 100 mg of PS daily, with a meal. Look for the trademarked Leci-PS™ from Lucas Meyer on the label of your favorite PS supplement manufacturer.

In addition, take 100 mg daily of DHA, with a meal. Look for the trademarked Neuromins™ from Martek Biosciences Corporation on the label of your favorite DHA supplement manufacturer.

### •In Support of Fatty Acids: ALC

Other noteworthy nutrients in building up the brain-immune connection fall in the category of amino acids. A number of important neurotransmitters associated with mental function and behavior are produced from certain amino acids, which can also act as neurotransmitters themselves.

Of all the amino acids, ALC (acetyl-L-carnitine) has been the one to receive most of the rave reviews for its essential role in transport and delivery of fatty acids into the cell. Once inside the cell membrane, fatty acids can then be used for energy metabolism and structural repair.

ALC is a naturally occurring amino acid found in meat and milk, and has demonstrated impressive success in protecting the brain from the ravages of aging. Currently, ALC is one of the most important natural substances under scientific scrutiny for its potential clinical applications in memory deficit disorders and maintaining memory in healthy individuals.

In human studies, ALC has been used over the past decade to treat Alzheimer's, with favorable results, and many studies document ALC's role in building up memory and the ability to perform problem-solving tasks.

While you must have an adequate intake of all the essential amino acids—and this is easily accomplished by consuming sufficient quantities of protein—later on in the book we will talk about manipulating the intake of individual amino acids in relation to treating specific brain diseases.

**RECOMMENDED DOSE FOR HEALTHY INDIVIDUALS:** 500 mg daily, on an empty stomach.

## The Second Foundation for Brain Health: Antioxidants and SAM

The brain's detoxifying mechanisms serve as the second foundation for health. These include the revolutionary new generation of antioxidants, the brain's best weapon against free radical damage, and S-adenosyl methionine (SAM).

## • Antioxidants that Protect the Brain: Your Best Weapon Against Toxic Free Radicals

As you will recall, with extra electrons available for donating, antioxidants can neutralize free radical attacks by satisfying the free radical quest for electrons. Antioxidants are especially important as we age, because they provide the best support against free radical damage to the body's time-weakened cellular structures and machinery.

During any challenge to your immune system—because of disease, infections, toxic exposure, stress, or aging—you need extra antioxidants to help scavenge the free radicals naturally produced by the immune system's cells during warfare.

As we discussed earlier, the brain's high fat content renders it especially vulnerable to free radicals, so the body has defined specific ways to protect brain cell fatty acids through special antioxidants. The special power of these antioxidants rests on their ability to cross the blood-brain barrier, the protective physical and chemical structure that surrounds the nervous system.

## • Glutathione

Glutathione is a naturally occurring amino acid that serves as an antioxidant with great detoxification powers, and the glutathione status of any cell is crucial to its health. Therefore, this natural, sulfur-containing peptide has a number of important roles to play in maintaining health and battling disease.

For one thing, glutathione is the major constituent of glutathione peroxidase, an antioxidant enzyme with crucial free radical—scavenging effects. Glutathione also plays a key role in keeping the body free of toxins by forming conjugates with a variety of toxic substances—including the deadly free radical, peroxynitrite.

What's more, glutathione is responsible for helping to maintain a proper oxidation state in the body. It does this by returning certain oxidized compounds back to their original forms—for example, turning oxidized vitamin C back to effective vitamin C.

Since glutathione is a major free radical scavenger in every cell, the loss of cellular glutathione has serious consequences to the life and death of that cell. Depressed glutathione levels are associated with the increased generation of free radicals found in Parkinson's patients, for example, and contributes to further brain cell death.

The best strategy for maintaining and producing sufficient cellular glutathione is to supplement the diet with n-acetyl-cysteine (NAC), selenium, and lipoic acid, which we discuss below. Studies have demonstrated that, when these nutrients are taken together, your body's cells are stimulated to increase natural glutathione production.

### • Lipoic Acid

Lipoic acid and vitamins C and E serve as the first line of defense against free radical damage. Unlike vitamin C, which is water-soluble, and vitamin E, which is fat-soluble, lipoic acid is a welcome wild card: it can act as a free radical scavenger in both fatty and water-filled components of the body.

Lipoic acid also has the ability to recycle other important antioxidants in the body, such as CE, glutathione, and coenzyme Q10. By working with the amino acid n-acetyl-cysteine (NAC), lipoic acid has the welcome potential to raise glutathione production (see below).

### • NAC (n-acetyl-cysteine)

A form of the amino acid cysteine, NAC is naturally produced by most living organisms and is well absorbed. In fact, NAC so readily crosses cell membranes and is so easily metabolized that only about 10 percent of the amount you consume stays in your blood for very long.

Clinicians have prescribed NAC for many years as an agent powerful enough to break up phlegm in the lungs, and a number of investigations have shown that NAC is particularly effective in detoxifying the body of toxic agents such as mercury, lead, environmental pollutants, and certain pesticides. More recently, NAC has been used as an antiviral agent and as an antioxidant in treating AIDS.

Currently, NAC is recognized for its role in stimulating cellular glutathione production, and serves as a useful adjunct nutrient in treating any illness warranting antioxidant therapy—a category that includes a number of different neurological diseases.

Along with lipoic acid, NAC is readily converted by the body to glutathione, the most important antioxidant and detoxifying system in every cell.

RECOMMENDED DAILY DOSAGES FOR HEALTHY INDIVIDUALS:

| | |
|---|---|
| NAC (n-acetyl-cysteine) | 500 mg, on an empty stomach |
| Lipoic acid | 100 mg, with food |
| Selenium | 200 mcg, with food (Do not exceed this amount.) |

## • Polyphenols: Avid Lipid Peroxidation Fighters

Antioxidants that fall into the polyphenol class (which includes bioflavonoids) demonstrate a wide variety of biochemical effects which can directly influence certain disease conditions.

One of the primary effects polyphenols have on the body is their greed for lipid peroxidation warfare: they're always ready to pair up with a free radical and calm it down. In addition, polyphenols spring into action when it becomes necessary to detoxify the body's blood of certain metals, such as iron, that may otherwise promote additional risky free radical activity if levels reach the danger mark.

Finally, polyphenols have a keen knack for slowing down the production of lipoxygenase, an enzyme that can turn up the heat under the body's inflammatory and allergic responses.

One interesting group of polyphenols, epigallocatechin gallate, is readily available through drinking green tea. This group has been studied by the American Health Foundation, which found it to be significantly better at inhibiting deadly peroxynitrite reactions than either vitamin C or glutathione.

Our own food supply is filled with polyphenols. Excellent dietary sources include red wine, green tea, berries and other fruits, soy beans, and dark vegetables. The best supplements include fruit polyphenols; grape seed extract; pine bark extract; Pycnogenol® (a special form of pine bark extract which contains a mixture of important polyphenolic components); and herbs such as bilberry, ginkgo, and milk thistle.

*RECOMMENDED DOSE FOR HEALTHY INDIVIDUALS:* 120 mg daily of either Pycnogenol®, fruit polyphenols or grape seed extract, or the same amount of a supplement that combines at least two into a single formula. Take these supplements with a meal.

## • The Tocopherols and Tocotrienols

One of the best-known antioxidants, vitamin E (tocopherol), is widely considered one of the most important fat soluble antioxidants to date. The rest of the story—which features the chemical relatives of tocopherols called tocotrienols—is only now beginning to unfold.

The tocotrienols, which are found predominantly in rice, bran, and rice or barley oil, have a unique chemical makeup that allows them to act as efficient free radical hunters by penetrating fatty acids effectively. Tocotrienols prevent oxidative damage of the fatty tissues that make up the brain.

*RECOMMENDED DOSES FOR HEALTHY INDIVIDUALS:* Since tocotrienols may prove to be better antioxidants than tocopherols, we suggest adding 50 mg of tocotrienols to your daily nutritional program. Additionally, we recommend taking 400 IUs of tocopherols. Take these supplements with a meal.

## • Coenzyme Q10.

Found in cell mitochondria, the antioxidant coenzyme Q10 plays a major role in cellular energy production. As you will learn in our chapters on Parkinson's disease and chronic fatigue syndrome, the mitochondria are organisms within all cells responsible for energy production, and are particularly vulnerable to free radical damage. Coenzyme Q10 is essential in defending them, because it is one of the few antioxidants that can actually penetrate mitochondria and provide a defense inside the mitochondrial membrane.

*RECOMMENDED DOSE FOR HEALTHY INDIVIDUALS:* 120 mg daily, taken with a meal.

## • SAM: Part of the Clean-up Crew

SAM (s-adenosyl methionine) is a substance that naturally occurs in all of your body's cells. Basically, SAM is a member of your body's clean-up crew, serving to detoxify cell membranes and synthesize neurotransmitters.

Besides clearing toxins out of your body, SAM enhances the body's own defense mechanisms by removing "used up" steroid hormones, thyroid hormones, and stale neurotransmitters, helping the body along when it's time to sweep harmful substances out the door.

In addition, SAM is one of the principal mediators when it comes to forming glutathione, the major cellular antioxidant. Depletion of glutathione is associated with aging and several neurological diseases. Because of its beneficial effects on raising intracellular glutathione levels, SAM is effective in treating liver disease and other conditions associated with chronic inflammation.

But that's not all this amazing substance can do: it is also a basic ingredient for building up strong cell membranes in the central nervous system.

Investigators have discovered that adding SAM to the diet of aging rats increases the number of acetylcholine receptor sites in the memory center of those rat brains—the hippocampal regions. Treating the rats with SAM increased the fluidity of cell membranes by stimulating phospholipid synthesis.

What's more, SAM has a beneficial effect on key neurotransmitters affecting mood, such as norepinephrine and serotonin. By increasing the ability of certain enzymes to synthesize norepinephrine and serotonin, SAM acts as a natural antidepressant without the side effects of prescription antidepressants currently on the market.

SAM has also proven effective in attention deficit disorder, perhaps because it increases the brain's production of catecholamines, the neurotransmitters we rely on to efficiently transmit nerve impulses.

**RECOMMENDED DOSE FOR HEALTHY INDIVIDUALS:** 200 mg daily, taken with a meal.

## • *Ginkgo Biloba: Leaves that Provide More than Shade*

The leaves of the ginkgo tree contain a number of important constituents. Researchers examining just how ginkgo biloba enhances our physiological functions have discovered that this natural compound has a number of wonderful properties. For example, it can:

- open the blood flow of arteries, veins, and capillaries.
- inhibit monamine oxidase, the enzyme that breaks down certain neurotransmitters in the brain.
- decrease the clumping of blood in vessels.
- increase cellular glucose uptake by hungry cells.
- act as a powerful antioxidant, protecting against lipid peroxidation and enhancing SOD activity.

Using ginkgo biloba in clinical trials, patients with a variety of disorders have experienced better health, such as improved blood flow, reduced dizziness, improved memory, and fewer headaches and depressive episodes. Thus, as you will see in the chapters that follow, ginkgo biloba extract is an essential ingredient in nutritional protocols for treating a variety of brain disorders.

RECOMMENDED DOSE FOR HEALTHY INDIVIDUALS: 60 mg daily of standardized ginkgo biloba extract, taken with a meal. Note: In order to provide a reliable and consistent dose of the active constituents found in ginkgo biloba, only purchase a *standardized* ginkgo biloba extract.

# The Third Foundation: The DHEA Hormone: The Best Answer to Too Much Cortisol

A steroid naturally produced by both your brain and adrenal glands, DHEA (dehydropiandrosterone) serves several important functions in the brain. For one thing, DHEA is essential for nurturing the growth and function of neuron dendrites, the tiny branching fibers that help brain cells stay in touch with one another and keep your brain's communication network in healthy working order. DHEA also promotes nutritional support within individual cells.

Your DHEA level peaks at adolescence and steadily declines as you age. However, you need DHEA just as much, or more, as time passes: DHEA protects you from the damaging effect of hormones produced by your body during times of stress—most notably, from the cortisol hormone we discussed in the previous chapter. DHEA actually buffers cells against the effects of overzealous cortisol activity, and partially regulates cortisol production.

As you may recall from our earlier chapter, cortisol is a hormone produced during stress that is currently under close scrutiny for its relationship to such diverse neurological diseases as depression and Alzheimer's. Investigators have determined that, when excess cortisol is produced as a result of stress, those high levels of cortisol can cause higher levels of free radicals and thus damage to healthy brain cells, particularly in regions of the brain responsible for memory and learning.

Additionally, human studies testing the effects of DHEA on the immune system have revealed that DHEA can normalize potentially dangerous cytokine levels. DHEA may prove especially beneficial in reeling in the cytokine interleukin 6, which has been linked to Alzheimer's.

> RECOMMENDED DOSE FOR HEALTHY INDIVIDUALS: People interested in adding a DHEA supplement should check with their health care practitioners about the appropriate use and dosage of DHEA for their individual needs.

## Conclusion

While ongoing animal and human studies continue to bring us new insights into the mechanisms by which nutrients and foods influence the brain–immune system connection, research in the emerging field of nutritional science has finally reached the patient bedside.

Today, we have the hard science to back up many theories in so-called "alternative" medicine that were once considered nothing more than old wives' tales or folklore by mainstream physicians and many patients. Just as there are nutrients that promote optimal health, we know with certainty that it is possible to use these neuroimmunomodulators as aggressive nutritional interventions in combination with mainstream medical and hormonal therapies to address specific illnesses.

As prevention becomes the focus of our evolving health care system, we can expect to continue refining nutritional protocols to maintain normal brain and immune system function in both healthy and compromised patients.

### TABLE 2

### SUPPLEMENTS FOR OPTIMAL BRAIN HEALTH

| Nutrient | Recommended Daily Doses |
|---|---|
| PS (Phosphatidylserine) | 100 mg, with a meal |
| DHA (Docosahexaneoic acid) | 100 mg, with a meal |
| Lipoic acid | 100 mg, with a meal |
| NAC (n-acetyl-cysteine) | 500 mg, on an empty stomach |
| Selenium* | 200 mcg, with a meal |
| Coenzyme Q10 | 120 mg, with a meal |
| Vitamin E (tocopherol/tocotrienol) | |
| Tocopherol | 400 IU |
| Tocotrienols | 50 mg, with a meal |
| Polyphenols | 60 mg, with a meal |
| (Pycnogenol®, grape seed extract, green tea extract, or fruit polyphenols.) | |
| Standardized ginkgo biloba extract | 60 mg, with a meal |

*If you are already taking selenium, avoid any amounts above 200 mcg.

# Treating Neurological Illnesses with Breakthrough Medical, Nutritional, and Immune-Boosting Therapies

# CHAPTER 5

# ALZHEIMER'S DISEASE

After her official retirement, Joan stayed on as a part-time consultant in the hospital public relations office where she had worked for over three decades. She enjoyed her job, and the extra money always came in handy. Besides, at sixty-nine she was still in good health and couldn't see the point of wasting all her time in the garden.

Gradually, though, she began to have trouble at work. At first it was the little things: She'd misfile a project, or forget the name of someone she knew in the next office. And one day she forgot her way to the cafeteria, where she'd been having lunch nearly every day since joining the staff.

Her coworkers began to tease her about being so forgetful. Joan made jokes right along with them, but she really wanted to cry. Wait until they got old and forgot things. They'd see how much fun it was.

Finally, one day Joan's supervisor suggested that perhaps it was time she took that retirement after all, and things seemed to go gradually downhill from there.

Joan's daughter brought her to the family doctor, but he dismissed her complaints as symptoms of the normal aging process.

A year went by, and things didn't get any better. Joan had difficulty sleeping, fumbled over routine daily tasks, and was hesitant about driving. She had to look at the daily newspaper to remember the date and kept forgetting the way to the supermarket. Worse still, she accused everyone in her family of hiding things in her house so she couldn't find them, and was so argumentative these days that her grandchildren grumbled about having to go there for Sunday dinners.

However, it wasn't until Joan took a walk one winter afternoon, wearing her best summer dress on a snowy day, that her family finally believed something was seriously wrong.

## Alzheimer's Disease: An Overview

Like more than 4 million Americans, Joan suffers from the beginning stages of Alzheimer's disease, the key cause of dementia among people over sixty-five.

The word "dementia" literally means "deprived of mind," and the primary effects of any dementia are cognitive. Over time, those with Alzheimer's experience a progressive loss of mental faculties, beginning with memory, learning, attention, and judgment—in short, all the activities that make us human.

While the symptoms of Alzheimer's in its early stages can mimic depression, psychosis, and various mental illnesses—sometimes causing physicians to make an erroneous early diagnosis—Alzheimer's is in fact a physical disorder whose symptoms are caused by the death and destruction of neurons in very specific areas of the brain.

People who have had Alzheimer's include many whose names you easily recognize, such as the illustrator Norman Rockwell, actress Rita Hayworth, essayist E. B. White, President Ronald Reagan, and film director Otto Preminger. For each of them, as for the people you know with Alzheimer's, the disease came at a devastating cost.

Without effective treatment, most people with Alzheimer's eventually become incapacitated. Experts estimate that about half of the nation's more than 1.3 million nursing home residents today may have Alzheimer's. More than 10 percent of people over sixty-five, and fully half of us who reach eighty-five, will suffer from the disease.

In fact, since being recognized early in the twentieth century as a distinct illness, Alzheimer's is being touted by some health care professionals as "the disease of the century," because we can expect to find a growing number of Alzheimer's patients in our population.

The reason is simple: Alzheimer's patients are predominantly over sixty-five years old, and Americans are living longer than ever before. People over eighty-five now make up the fastest-growing age group in the United States, and the Census Bureau predicts that 5.1 million Americans will be over eighty-five by the year 2000, compared to just 2.5 million in that category in 1982. By the year 2034, we can expect to see three times as many people with Alzheimer's disease as we find in our population today.

About seven out of every ten Alzheimer's patients live with their families, and the emotional, physical, and financial burdens those families suffer are enormous.

The caretakers of Alzheimer's patients are often the hidden victims of the disease. Besides watching the people they love become increasingly forgetful, confused, and unable to function on their own, family members of Alzheimer's patients face the painful task of deciding how to care for their loved ones over the long term. Whether an Alzheimer's patient lives at home or in a nursing home, the cost can reach upwards of $47,000 annually—an enormous economic burden to both family and society.

Though we have no cure as yet for Alzheimer's, we have come a long way in understanding some of its possible causes, the abnormalities in the brain underlying the symptoms of Alzheimer's, and ways to slow its progression.

From onset of symptoms to diagnosis, from treatment to hope on the horizon, in this chapter we will discuss Alzheimer's disease in the context of some of the most exciting—and effective—hormonal and nutritional therapies available today. These therapies truly do offer hope to Alzheimer's patients and their families, alleviating disease symptoms by treating chemical imbalances in the brain-immune connection.

The focus of the nutritional therapy we describe here is directed at:

1. Improving memory, language, reasoning, and judgment by providing supplementary compounds that assist with the synthesis and release of neurotransmitters.
2. Reducing the production of cellular toxins in the brain brought on by inadvertent or excessive activation of the immune system.
3. Slowing or stopping oxidative damage to cells.

In addition to discussing medical interventions, we will offer you a blueprint for a rigorous, progressive treatment plan which includes medical therapies, hormonal interventions, standardized herb extracts, and vitamins.

As with any therapeutic approach, this multifaceted treatment strategy is most successful when instituted in the early stages of the disease. Additionally, we urge anyone with a family history of Alzheimer's to participate in this diet and supplement program as a preventive measure.

## What Goes Wrong in Alzheimer's, and Why?

Almost everything we know about Alzheimer's has come from examining the brains of patients who died of the disease and generously donated their organs to science. Looking at one of these brains provides a visual clue to the biology of the disease: the sulci, or valleys between the brain tissue that give the brain its wrinkled appearance, are distinctly wider in the brain of a person with Alzheimer's than they are in healthy brains.

Alzheimer's was first discovered in 1906 by Alois Alzheimer, who observed unusual changes in the brain of a woman who died at age fifty-five, five years after developing dementia. Using special silver stains to more clearly reveal the structure of this woman's brain cells, Alzheimer discovered that the cerebral cortex—the seat of our intellectual functions—contained abnormal nerve cells with tangled fibers and clusters of degenerating nerve endings.

In Alzheimer's disease, the intricate process of communication between nerve cells is derailed owing to loss of connections between nerve cells brought on by neuron dysfunction and the death of neurons. The disease primarily strikes the hippocampus, a structure deep in the brain that is involved with cognition and memory.

## 1. *A New Gene Provides Clues*

Genes are biologic units located on chromosomes, structures in the nucleus of each cell. Genes transmit hereditary information using the molecule DNA (deoxyribonucleic acid). We now know that even the slightest alterations in the DNA code can produce a faulty protein—and those faulty proteins can lead to cellular weakening or breakdown.

Today's Alzheimer's researchers have linked one gene alteration in particular to the neuron dysfunction leading to Alzheimer's. It involves the apolipoprotein-E, or ApoE, gene, which helps transport cholesterol through the human body and form healthy cellular membranes for the brain's neurons. We all have ApoE, but whether we are susceptible to Alzheimer's or not largely depends on which version of this gene we inherited from our parents: ApoE2, ApoE3, or ApoE4.

Genetic research reveals that people who inherit the gene which encodes for ApoE4 have the highest chance of getting Alzheimer's.

Recently, for example, researchers at the Duke University General Clinical Research Center and the Joseph and Kathleen Bryan Alzheimer's Disease Research Center in Durham, North Carolina, collaborated on studies linking the ApoE4 gene and Alzheimer's. They discovered that the risk for Alzheimer's for people with copies of the ApoE4 gene from both parents is *three times greater* than that for other people.

Meanwhile, scientists at the Mayo Clinic in Rochester, Minnesota, chose to follow a group of older patients who suffered mild memory impairment. They found that over two-thirds of the patients who developed clinical dementia had a copy of the gene for ApoE4, and concluded that the presence of ApoE4 was the best predictor for Alzheimer's.

### 2. *Faulty ApoE Genes Impair Healthy Cell Membranes*

Just why is a defective ApoE gene linked to Alzheimer's?

Recent studies at the McGill Center for Studies in Aging in Quebec, Canada, suggest that the ApoE gene plays a central role in how effectively the brain's hippocampus responds to injury, particularly when it comes to regulating the transport of the cholesterol and phospholipids so crucial to building strong neuron membranes.

Although we have not yet pinpointed every step of the Alzheimer's pathology, we do know that people who inherit a certain mutation of the ApoE gene are, in effect, getting a faulty version of this otherwise helpful protein. They are therefore missing out on the building blocks of fat so essential to building up healthy cell membranes.

### 3. *Protein Plaques Form on the Brain*

In Alzheimer's patients, researchers have discovered plaques, or patches of dead cells and other castoff material, lying outside the brain's neurons. Most of these plaques are located in the areas of the brain associated with memory.

At the core of each of these plaques is a potentially deadly substance called beta amyloid, an abnormal protein not usually found in the brain.

Beta amyloid is a protein chopped off from a larger parent molecule known as amyloid precursor protein, or APP, during regular cellular metabolism.

In a recent paper published in *The New England Journal of Medicine,* Harvard Medical School researchers explain that APP is normally inserted partially into the membrane, and then the protruding part is cleaved, releasing a soluble form of the precursor protein. That way, an intact beta amyloid peptide is not normally generated. Production of the beta amyloid peptide in the aging brain, or in the brain affected by Alzheimer's, requires a change in the normal processing of APP which, in turn, results in abnormally high levels of beta amyloid.

How do increased levels of the beta amyloid protein contribute to the cascade of steps ultimately resulting in neuron death?

Investigators believe that neurons in the hippocampus die when beta amyloid is added, leading to the hypothesis that this protein is toxic to neurons when freed from its parent substance. In other words, beta amyloid breaks into pieces and sends out free radicals, the unstable molecules that can do the body so much damage.

In summary, then, people who inherit the defective ApoE4 gene have neurons that are inherently less structurally sound and may die more easily. This cell death sets off an immune response characterized by an increased production of fighter white blood cells and their chemical clearing tools to remove castoff fragments of dead or dying nerve cells at the site of injury.

In patients with Alzheimer's, beta amyloid may be viewed by the body as a toxic invader initially responsible for killing off mature neurons and causing further damage to neuron cell membranes. The immune system responds to the accumulation of damage accordingly.

As the plaques form, the immune system's messengers, the cytokines, amplify the body's response. In particular, the immune system calls upon a cytokine known as interleukin-6, which has the power to cleave APP, the amyloid precursor protein, thus releasing beta amyloid and damaging vulnerable neurons.

If, indeed, it is true that the neurons of Alzheimer's patients are being killed off as a direct consequence of beta amyloid, new research efforts will focus on developing certain drugs which may act as amyloid protease inhibitors. We hope someday to develop therapies that successfully block the production of this toxic protein and thus alleviate the symptoms of Alzheimer's.

### 4. *The Brain's Ability to Produce Acetylcholine is Impaired*

Ultimately, then, the brain's neurons die off in Alzheimer's disease owing to the effects of beta amyloid and free radicals. The brain region of greatest injury appears to be in the hippocampus's nucleus basalis of Mynert, the brain's central processing plant for the neurotransmitter acetylcholine.

Acetylcholine is the chemical essential for communication

### TABLE 3

## WHAT CAUSES ALZHEIMER'S?

- A defective apolipoprotein-E gene (ApoE4) is inherited.

- This defective gene causes ineffective synthesis of cell membranes responsible for protecting the brain's neurons from injury.

- An inadvertent, overzealous immune system response occurs owing to faulty cell membranes.

- The immune system messenger cytokine, interleukin-6, is overproduced.

- Increased levels of interleukin-6 stimulate beta amyloid to break off from its parent molecule, amyloid precursor protein (APP).

- Beta amyloid causes free radical injury to cells, promoting neuron death in the area of the brain responsible for producing acetylcholine, a neurotransmitter essential for memory and cognition.

between neurons responsible for memory and cognitive thinking. When acetylcholine levels fall dramatically, we see the memory loss and faulty reasoning that are hallmark symptoms of Alzheimer's.

## What About Environmental Suspects in Alzheimer's?

Although researchers have studied a number of environmental suspects as causal factors in Alzheimer's disease—particularly zinc and aluminum—the scientific community is still debating the effects of these elements. While zinc is an essential mineral that plays numerous roles in health and disease, it may be negatively associated with Alzheimer's disease.

The theory that using aluminum cookware or drinking water

treated with aluminum may be a risk factor dates back to the 1970s, when scientists first discovered traces of aluminum and iron in the brain plaques of people with Alzheimer's. Subsequent studies since then have produced conflicting results, however.

While researchers at the Mount Sinai School of Medicine's Department of Pathology were able to use atomic absorption spectrometry to show that the diseased brain tissue of certain Alzheimer's patients had a two- to three-fold increase in aluminum, others have demonstrated that groups of people exposed to unnaturally high levels of aluminum show no increased risk of Alzheimer's.

Nevertheless, aluminum is a neurotoxin that can impair cognition, and has been found to interfere with more than fifty neurochemical reactions. Because of this, and because brain aluminum levels are increased in patients with Alzheimer's, it would be sensible to avoid as much aluminum as possible. From aluminum cookware to aluminum-based deodorants and antacids, we encourage you to read labels and make educated choices.

Zinc has also been linked to Alzheimer's in controversial ways. Some scientists suggest that too little zinc is at fault, while others hypothesize that too much zinc can contribute to neuron death by causing soluble beta amyloid from the cerebrospinal fluid to form clumps similar to Alzheimer's plaques. There are other studies that do link a zinc deficiency with the symptoms of Alzheimer's.

In short then, we can say this: The jury is still out on the link between aluminum and zinc levels and Alzheimer's disease. We can expect investigations to continue in both of those areas in the decade to come.

# A Complete Blueprint for Care

Slowing the progression of Alzheimer's disease is dependent on saving the brain's acetylcholine-producing neurons from untimely deterioration and death and boosting both memory and cognitive function to improve quality of life.

Here, we describe a complete nutritional, hormonal, and medical protocol for aggressively treating patients with Alzheimer's. This protocol includes the latest recommendations for incorporating neuroimmunomodulators into your therapy.

## When Should You Suspect Alzheimer's?

Both for those afflicted with the disease and for the people who care for them, Alzheimer's is one of the most heartbreaking diseases known to mankind. When untreated, the disease eventually impairs all aspects of thought, feeling, and behavior, and carries a sentence of eventual mental emptiness imposed anywhere from ten months to ten years after onset.

Not all symptoms are present consistently or concurrently. While a cardinal feature of Alzheimer's disease is memory loss, early symptoms may also include changes in personality, speech difficulty, and errors in perception and judgment.

Initially, Alzheimer's victims may become withdrawn or lose interest in activities they used to enjoy—leading some family members and physicians to believe the person is suffering from clinical depression. Indeed, the two diseases have a strong association, which we will discuss later.

Additionally, Alzheimer's patients may have trouble recalling recently acquired information, while their long-term memories remain preserved. Misplacing objects and missing appointments are two cues for this stage of the disease.

People with Alzheimer's may exhibit paranoid behavior as the disease progresses. For example, a husband might accuse his wife of cheating on him, or a grandmother who lives alone might believe someone is sneaking into her house and rearranging things. Typically, the person you know with Alzheimer's will also have sleep disturbances, waking up in the middle of the night to get dressed and carry out activities as if it were daytime.

In later stages of Alzheimer's, language difficulties may become insurmountable, beginning with difficulty in recalling the names of objects or family members, and progressing to the point where people with Alzheimer's produce completely meaningless sentences.

In advanced stages of Alzheimer's, patients may become completely bedridden, regressed, and unable to perform even life's most basic tasks, such as getting dressed or feeding themselves.

## Diagnosing Alzheimer's: Seeing Behind the Masks

As with most diseases, the earlier Alzheimer's is diagnosed, the better our chances are of using aggressive therapies to slow its progress.

Because Alzheimer's mimics so many other disorders, the disease can wear many masks. It's crucial to see behind those masks in order to make a correct diagnosis. There is no single laboratory test we can perform to diagnose the disease.

We stress that anyone who suspects Alzheimer's in themselves or in a loved one because of the symptoms described above should see a qualified neurologist to rule out other common—and often treatable—causes of similar symptoms.

Some of the other disorders that may masquerade as Alzheimer's include:

*Ministrokes.* The second most common cause of dementia, multi-infarct dementia, is a consequence of brain damage caused by a series of small strokes or injuries to blood vessels in the brain. Ministrokes are different from Alzheimer's in that the damage is localized to one side of the body and the dementia progresses in rapid steps, rather than along the steady ramp of decline experienced by those with Alzheimer's. Ministrokes can be detected by a CAT scan or MRI scan of the brain.

*Visual and hearing impairment.* Because elderly patients are particularly vulnerable to declining sensory function, it's important to rule this out as a cause for your loved one's perceptual errors. Adequate hearing and visual evaluations can determine whether the person simply needs corrective lenses or a hearing aid to improve function.

*Depression.* We will discuss the etiology of clinical depression later in this book. Here, it is important to note that depression is often referred to as "pseudodementia" because mood changes can significantly affect how a person behaves. Depression can produce poor concentration, withdrawn behavior, and forgetfulness—all of which can be addressed through nutritional therapies and antidepressants.

*Drug use.* As older people are often being treated with pharmacological compounds for other illnesses or injuries, it's important to rule out possible side effects of drug use before arriving at an Alzheimer's diagnosis. Compounds which most easily cause Alzheimer's-like symptoms include minor tranquilizers, certain heart drugs, and substances known as anticholinergics, all of which may cause memory problems. (Note: Never discontinue any medication on your own without consulting your physician.)

*Vitamins B12 and B1 deficiency.* As we noted in earlier chapters, vitamin deficiencies have been the culprits for many a disease. We now have virtually indisputable evidence that all of the B vitamins play critical roles in brain health, but we place an added value on the benefits of thiamine (B1) and cobalamin (B12).

For people with Alzheimer's, it is essential that a vitamin B deficiency be ruled out, as many symptoms of a vitamin B deficiency mimic Alzheimer's symptoms—yet are readily treated by increasing the individual's intake of B vitamins.

In addition, there may be a relationship between Alzheimer's and vitamin B deficiency as well. Several studies, for example, have pointed to low levels of vitamin B12 in the cerebrospinal fluid of Alzheimer's patients. In 1990, researchers from the Yamaguchi University School of Medicine in Japan found that patients with Alzheimer's disease had significantly lower cerebrospinal fluid vitamin B12 levels than patients suffering multi-infarct dementia.

Researchers in various medical centers have discovered that patients with Alzheimer's have significantly lower plasma thiamine levels than control patients. In addition, the improper metabolism of thiamine in Alzheimer's patients may result in a deficiency of the important thiamine diphosphate molecule in the brain, impairing the ability to think. In one study reported in the *Annals of Neurology,* Alzheimer's patients treated with thiamine improved their cognitive abilities.

Unfortunately, many times test results show vitamin B levels which would not automatically arouse suspicion of a deficiency. Adequate blood levels of nutrients very often do not reflect tissue stores. It is necessary to run additional tests to diagnose the problem. One specific type of blood test, known as a measurement of homocysteine, may be a much more sensitive index of subclinical B12 deficiency.

*Sleep disorder.* One of the most common but frequently overlooked contributors to memory disorder in the elderly is the fact that some people have a great deal of trouble sleeping as they age. One condition, known as sleep apnea, is associated with forgetfulness, high blood pressure, and falling asleep at odd times during the day. Sleep apnea can contribute to both dementia and hypertension. One clue to its appearance is snoring at night.

## Nutritional Therapies You Should Begin Incorporating Now

Once your neurologist has determined that you or your loved one is suffering from Alzheimer's, there are a number of nutritional supplements you can immediately—and safely—incorporate into your diet.

The focus of nutritional therapy for Alzheimer's patients is on improving memory, language, reasoning, and judgment by assisting with the synthesis and release of neurotransmitters, increasing blood flow, reducing the production of amyloid via interleukin-6, and slowing or stopping the progression of oxidative damage to the brain.

These goals may be accomplished through nutritional therapy in combination with medical and hormonal interventions. The nutritional therapy includes supplements, standardized herb extracts, and hormone balancing.

The nutritional compounds we have found to be of the most benefit in slowing or even halting the progress of Alzheimer's are vitamin E, ALC (acetyl-L-carnitine), PS, and DHA.

Additionally, we recommend that patients consider taking antioxidants and ginkgo biloba supplements. All these agents are under examination for their potential as neuroimmunomodulators, and show promise in alleviating the symptoms of memory loss and problems in cognitive thinking, thus improving the quality of life for Alzheimer's patients.

All of these nutritional agents are readily available by themselves—and are safe to take over the counter in the dosages recommended below. These compounds show no evidence of interacting with other medications in any negative way.

One more compound, CDP choline, is currently being examined worldwide for its potential neuroimmunomodulating benefits in treating Alzheimer's, and may become available by prescription in the United States pending further studies.

## The First Step to Take: Begin a Healthy Diet

One of the first steps Alzheimer's patients can take toward halting the progression of the disease is to adjust their diets to observe the basic guidelines outlined in Chapter 3 for feeding the brain-immune connection.

## Add ALC (Acetyl-L-Carnitine) to Counteract Cellular Breakdown

ALC is a natural substance derived from the amino acid L-carnitine, and works with L-carnitine to help fatty acids cross into inner mitochondrial membranes.

In 1996, a multicenter study was conducted by researchers at the University of California, New York University, and Columbia Presbyterian Hospital with 450 patients with Alzheimer's disease to determine the effectiveness of treating those patients with ALC. In this landmark investigation, researchers found that the majority of patients who were under sixty-five years old and were taking ALC demonstrated significant reduction in their rate of decline when compared to patients taking placebos.

Why is ALC a beneficial nutrient for Alzheimer's patients? Of particular interest to scientists and clinicians is the fact that ALC is structurally similar to acetylcholine, the memory neurotransmitter. In fact, ALC displays similar actions in the central nervous system both directly and through its supportive effect on choline acetyltransferase, the enzyme we count on for acetylcholine synthesis and release.

ALC is an active antioxidant and protects the cell membranes of neurons against free radical attacks. In addition, ALC promotes phospholipid metabolism and enhances brain energy production.

Since investigators have already implicated abnormal energy processing as a culprit of cell death and cell membrane disruption in Alzheimer's, they theorize that ALC's benefits may extend far beyond its ability to influence the way our brains produce acetylcholine.

Additionally, ALC counteracts the age-dependent reduction of several receptors in the central nervous system of animals, including receptors for neurotransmitters and nerve growth factor.

In one study, for example, 2.5 grams of ALC administered daily for three months helped Alzheimer's patients perform better on a variety of cognitive tasks. Investigators concluded that ALC may retard dementia, particularly in patients suffering only mild to moderate symptoms of Alzheimer's.

ALC is a safe, effective treatment that should be part of the therapeutic protocol for anyone with Alzheimer's disease.

RECOMMENDED DOSE: Anyone diagnosed with Alzheimer's should immediately begin taking ALC supplements of 2 g daily between meals.

## PS (Phosphatidylserine): The Mason of Cell Membranes

The first step in treating patients with Alzheimer's disease is to rebuild defective cell membranes. As you already know, neuron membranes are made up primarily of different lipids, or fats.

The brain's major phospholipids are key to providing cell membranes with "fluidity," the ability to allow various substances to pass in and out of the cell. As you can guess, this property is essential to the cell-to-cell "talk" carried on by neurotransmitters.

Our brain health depends on one major phospholipid, or

fatty acid, in particular, phosphatidylserine (PS), for a number of important metabolic effects. Besides making it possible for nutrients to move freely in and out of neurons, PS is necessary for cells to metabolize energy-essential glucose. PS also helps cells protect themselves from lethal free radicals on a blitzkrieg through our bodies as a result of the overboard immune response associated with Alzheimer's.

When researchers at the Vanderbilt University School of Medicine and Memory Study studied PS in clinical trials, they found that taking PS orally helped patients with Alzheimer's improve memory, learning, and cognitive functions. Not surprisingly, differences in PS-treated groups versus the placebo groups in that study were most apparent among patients in the early stages of Alzheimer's.

In further support of the benefits of PS as a neuroimmunomodulator, investigators who conducted a multicenter study with over 140 patients found that those who took PS showed significant improvement on cognitive tests. Even after treatment stopped, the group that had received PS sustained improvement, leading those investigators to hypothesize that PS produces structural changes in cell membranes rather than transient metabolic changes.

Today, PS is available from soy lecithin extract in 100 mg softgels. It is interesting to note that the bovine extract used in the study described above may have contained other important neuronutrients, such as the omega-3 fatty acids docosahexanoic acid (DHA) which we discuss below.

RECOMMENDED DOSE: Patients diagnosed with Alzheimer's should incorporate a supplement of 300 mg of PS, taken with a meal, into their daily nutrients. Look for the trademarked Leci-PS™ from Lucas Meyer.

## DHA (Docosahexanoic Acid): Monitoring Calcium Across Cell Walls

The primary phospholipid component of the cell membranes surrounding neurons is DHA, a structural fatty acid. Compared to other organs, in fact, the brain has an unusually high content of lipids. Even limited alterations in lipid structure or amount may be of considerable importance, as those alterations may affect the way that membranes pass neurotransmitters and other chemicals in and out of cells.

Many researchers believe that changes in the composition and metabolism of fatty acids like DHA may contribute to Alzheimer's. In one major Swedish study, investigators demonstrated that the brain DHA content of Alzheimer's patients was significantly less than the levels in the brains of control patients.

Additionally, researchers believe that DHA is a primary player when it comes to monitoring how much calcium crosses neuronal membranes. Owing to its unusual chemical structure, DHA has the ability to block calcium channels in the cell.

Why is DHA's role as a calcium channel blocker so important? Basically, in disease conditions where the amount of DHA is decreased, as in Alzheimer's, research has shown that cellular calcium levels are elevated. When calcium enters a cell, it activates a protease enzyme which can convert the large APP molecule we discussed earlier into beta amyloid, the toxic protein found in Alzheimer's plaques.

Today DHA, which was commonly found in fish oils, may be purchased by itself. Essentially it is DHA, not EPA, that is important for brain health. Commonly found in fish oil products, we recommend taking supplements of DHA in the preferred vegetarian algae form (Neuromins™).

RECOMMENDED DOSE: 300 mg daily, taken with a meal. Look for the trademarked Neuromins™ from Martek Biosciences Corporation.

## CDP: A Communication Facilitator

Scientists perceived long ago that choline phospholipids also serve as important components of cell membranes. In fact, without an adequate supply of choline, neurons cannot transmit messages across synapses, fall short when it comes to manufacturing enough of the acetylcholine neurotransmitter, and are prevented from synthesizing phosphatidylcholine as well.

Now, new studies provide additional hope for Alzheimer's patients diagnosed in the later stages of the disease. By using a form of choline called CDP (cytidine diphosphate choline), scientists have discovered that they can provoke the brain to manufacture more acetylcholine. CDP choline can also increase the amounts of phospholipids in brain membranes.

For instance, in a study published in the *Annals of the New York Academy of Sciences,* Spanish investigators reported patients with Alzheimer's disease treated with a daily dose of 1,000 mg per day of CDP for one month showed a modest improvement in mental performance. They hypothesized that CDP choline may contribute to neuron membrane repair, bestow a moderate antidepressant effect, and slow the overactive immune response by reducing serum interleukin-1B levels, particularly in patients in the early stages of Alzheimer's.

> *RECOMMENDED DOSE:* Check with your physician to find out when CDP choline will become available in the U.S. market. Meanwhile, patients with Alzheimer's should ensure they are receiving adequate choline. We recommend taking 4 g of choline with a meal, either as phosphatidylcholine (PC) or as a combination of PC and choline bitartrate or choline chloride.

## Antioxidants: Keeping Free Radicals Under Control

As researchers understand more about how we age, one thing has become abundantly clear: One of the most significant reasons people age is our cells' increasing inability to fight off destructive oxygen free radicals.

As you already know from reading our earlier chapters, when the body's immune system mobilizes, our cells metabolize more oxygen and spin off by-products called oxygen free radicals. These free radicals destroy invaders efficiently. Unfortunately, they can also rampage through the body and attack our own cells, chewing through cellular membranes and attacking the very DNA that contains cellular genetic codes.

Alzheimer's patients suffer from higher than normal levels of free radicals. Recently, Canadian scientists discovered that samples of Alzheimer's brain tissue produced nearly 50 percent more free radicals than did controls. Studies like this one lead investigators to conclude that there is great promise for Alzheimer's patients in the potential of antioxidants to help reduce the inflammation and inadvertent cell death caused by the body's own immune system's oxidative stress on cells.

In particular, clinicians and researchers are now examining the possible protective effects of fat-soluble antioxidants against free radicals, as these are able to cross the blood-brain barrier and enter the regions of the brain where they are most desperately needed.*

RECOMMENDED DOSE: We recommend that Alzheimer's patients take an advanced multiple antioxidant supplement containing a complete array of the most important antioxidant nutrients, especially the fat-soluble ones. These include coenzyme Q10, vitamin E, tocotrienols, and carotenoids (including alpha and beta carotene, lutein, lycopene, and zeaxanthin). Patients should follow the dosages suggested on the labels.

Additional beneficial antioxidants include lipoic acid, n-acetyl-cysteine (NAC), and vitamin C. Essentially, you can obtain the majority of antioxidants by looking for an advanced antioxidant formula. Additionally, patients with Alzheimer's need to add 200 mg of coenzyme Q10, 200 mg of lipoic acid, 500 mg of NAC, and 120 mg of Pycnogenol®, grape seed or fruit polyphenols, since many formulas do not contain these therapeutic quantities. All these supplements are to be taken with a meal.

---

*A recent study which appeared in the *New England Journal of Medicine* supports the connection between free radicals and Alzheimer's Disease. Alzheimer's patients treated with high doses of vitamin E and selegiline were demonstrated to have a significant delay in progression of cognitive impairment.

## Important Accessory Nutrients for Alzheimer's Patients

### • *Ginkgo biloba standardized extract: Increasing Blood Flow*

Decreased blood flow to the brain plays a major role in age-related brain disorders. Now, clinicians are employing ginkgo biloba extracts to increase blood flow and decrease free radical damage in the brain.

The active components of ginkgo extracts are found in ginkgo-flavoglycosides and terpene lactones, compounds which affect the brain's ability to inhibit the breakdown of certain neurotransmitters and enhance the release of others.

Scientists have used ginkgo extracts in addressing symptoms such as memory loss, dizziness, and depression. For Alzheimer's patients, a study conducted at the Universitat Berlin in Germany holds particular promise: Researchers there conducted a double-blind, placebo-controlled trial with 216 patients, and discovered that patients treated with 240 mg of ginkgo biloba daily showed fewer symptoms of dementia than patients in the control group. In addition, ginkgo has been found to be a very potent free radical scavenger of superoxide and peroxyl radicals and protects fatty cell membranes from oxidation.

RECOMMENDED DOSE: 240 mg daily of standardized ginkgo biloba extract.

## What Other Neuroimmunomodulators Should You Discuss with Your Doctor?

In addition to adding the nutritional supplements we describe above, anyone diagnosed with Alzheimer's should discuss hormone and anti-inflammatory therapies with a physician, as these have also proven to be of great neuroimmunomodulating benefit to anyone with Alzheimer's.

Your personal health care practitioner can recommend the best doses of these hormones for you and weigh the risks against benefits, given your individual medical history.

## Hormone Therapies

As you may recall from Chapter 1, "Brain-Immune Connection Basics," the immune system's cytokines serve as advanced scouts, heralding a cry for more soldiers. Sometimes, these cytokines amplify the immune response beyond what is needed, causing detrimental effects to healthy cells.

One cytokine in particular, interleukin-6, has the ability to turn a helpful response into a potentially destructive one by unleashing the damaging effects of beta amyloid, a toxic substance found in the brains of people with Alzheimer's disease. Factors that reduce the production of interleukin-6 can potentially inhibit the synthesis of beta amyloid.

One substance with the potential to inhibit amyloid synthesis is estrogen—but its use as a therapy for Alzheimer's patients is a controversial one.

As reported in Harvard Medical School's *Women's Health Watch* in November 1996, estrogen's influence on cognitive function has been an intriguing area of research recently. In particular, estrogen seems to be an important player in preserving the brain's choligeneric neurons—the cells most affected in Alzheimer's disease—and in nourishing the hippocampus, the part of the brain so pivotal to good memory.

The high incidence of Alzheimer's among postmenopausal women suggests that, as estrogen levels fall, women are increasingly vulnerable to Alzheimer's disease. This idea is supported by a number of observations.

For instance, Dr. Brenner and his colleagues reported in a recent issue of the *American Journal of Epidemiology* that women taking estrogen were less likely to have Alzheimer's than those who did not. Scientists at the University of Southern California and other medical centers nationwide have also revealed that postmenopausal estrogen replacement therapy may be beneficial in decreasing the risk of Alzheimer's.

It may be that estrogen plays a protective role owing to its ability to inhibit the production of interleukin-6, the cytokine which can have such a devastating effect on prodding the immune system to turn against brain cells.

How does estrogen protect against Alzheimer's? While we

have not pinpointed its effects entirely, researchers believe that estrogen may help maintain nerve growth factor, which we know stimulates and maintains the integrity of the brain's neurons. Furthermore, estrogen may also promote the production of an enzyme necessary for the body to synthesize acetylcholine in the brain.

With so many studies outlining the beneficial effects of estrogen in treating Alzheimer's, where do our concerns lie?

Primarily, recent research suggests that women using estrogen may put themselves at greater risk for women's cancers, and for breast cancer in particular. Therefore, women who are considering adding estrogen to their Alzheimer's therapies should consult their physicians and think carefully about their own family histories. A personal or family history of breast cancer, an undiagnosed lump in the breast, or possibly even the presence of fibrocystic disease should all be contraindications to taking estrogen.

## Soy Isoflavones: An Alternative to Estrogen

Due to the controversy surrounding estrogen replacement therapy, we strongly suggest that patients explore the possibility of alternative natural approaches to influencing the body's estrogen production.

One of these is to add soybeans and soy foods to the diet, as these foods contain a group of interesting compounds called isoflavones. Isoflavones are natural plant phytoestrogens and have several beneficial effects on human health, including regulating hormone balance and providing protection against cancer and heart disease.

Chemically, isoflavones look like estrogen and are converted to form very weak estrogens in the body. Despite being weak in the negative effects associated with estrogen, they are potent protective compounds in the body and play an important role in estrogen replacement therapy.

While soy is not the only plant source of isoflavones, it is one of the richest sources, especially of genistein—the most studied of the isoflavones. We recommend that patients with Alzheimer's add genistein as well as a general soy isoflavone concentrate to their diets.

RECOMMENDED DOSE: 100 mg of isoflavone concentrate daily and 60 mg of genistein, both taken with a meal. Look for isoflavone concentrates with high levels of genistein. Additionally, there are high isoflavone soy protein powders available.

## Anti-inflammatory Agents: Fighting Off Attacks by Our Own Immune Systems

As we have already discussed, inflammatory changes in the brains of Alzheimer's patients may be caused by various types of immune system attacks brought on by the presence of the toxic beta amyloid protein. Anti-inflammatory agents may therefore be therapeutic in Alzheimer's patients by reducing this destructive immune activity.

For instance, investigators reported in an August 1993 issue of *Neurology* that administering 100 to 150 mg per day of indomethacin, a nonsteroidal anti-inflammatory substance, was beneficial in protecting Alzheimer's patients from cognitive decline.

This data, when taken together with retrospective data on patients taking nonsteroidals, suggests that anti-inflammatory drugs may protect people with Alzheimer's from suffering so much immune-mediated damage.

Unfortunately, nonsteroidals are frequently associated with gastrointestinal bleeding, especially in elderly patients. A safer, nontoxic strategy may involve the use of antioxidants, omega-3 fatty acids, and polyphenols, all of which we described earlier.

## Additional Medical Therapies to Discuss with Your Health Care Provider

Researchers are currently investigating just how the cholinergic pathways in the cerebral cortex and basal forebrain are compromised in Alzheimer's patients. Others are working toward developing drugs that can enhance the surviving cholinergic system, protecting the neurons that produce acetylcholine from further damage.

The most widely investigated drugs for treating Alzheimer's so far are the cholinesterase (ChE) inhibitors. These have the potential to increase the concentration of acetylcholine for synaptic transmission by inhibiting the enzymes guilty of breaking acetylcholine down and rendering it useless.

One ChE inhibitor to have received the widest attention of late is Donepezil. Donepezil is chemically distinct from other ChE inhibitors, and has been developed specifically for treating Alzheimer's disease. In preclinical studies, Donepezil has proved to be useful in selectively inhibiting ChE in brain tissue and slowing the decline in memory among patients with Alzheimer's.

## Putting It All Together

Once Joan was diagnosed with Alzheimer's disease, we immediately recommended that she add supplements of ALC (acetyl-L-carnitine), PS (phosphatidylserine) and DHA to her diet, as well as asking her daughter to help Joan increase her consumption of antioxidants and fatty fish such as tuna, salmon, etc.

In addition, we encouraged Joan to continue exercising her mind through activities she normally enjoyed but had begun to give up in frustration. These activities include crossword puzzles, reading the newspaper, and gardening. In each case, we make certain that she sets goals and is supervised by a family member or home health aide in reaching them.

During the past year, Joan has returned to her neurologist for follow-ups every three months. Although her underlying memory impairments remain, Joan has shown little progression in her Alzheimer's symptoms and is still largely able to care for herself. Her family, meanwhile, has joined one of the support groups for Alzheimer's listed at the end of this book—an important step in helping everyone understand and manage Joan's disease.

Now that you have an overview of Alzheimer's disease and how it affects the very structure, function, and biochemical metabolism of our brain-immune system connection, you are probably eager to get started—or to help someone you love begin—investigating a complete neuroimmunomodulating treatment protocol. Here is our own summary guideline for treatment.

*Preventive Strategies*

> Estrogen (taken only under the supervision of a health care practitioner)
> Indomethacin and other nonsteroidal anti-inflammatories
> Selegiline (by prescription)

*Daily Nutritional Supplements*

| | |
|---|---|
| ALC (acetyl-L-carnitine) | 2 g, on an empty stomach |
| PS (Leci-PS™ phosphatidylserine) | 300 mg, with food |
| DHA (Neuromins™ docosahexanoic acid) | 300 mg, with food |
| Choline | 4 g, with food |
| Antioxidants | A complete antioxidant supplement, taken in the amounts prescribed by the formula label |
| Coenzyme Q10 | 200 mg, with food |
| Lipoic acid | 200 mg, with food |
| NAC (n-acetyl-cysteine) | 1 g, on an empty stomach |
| Ginkgo biloba | 240 mg, standardized extract with food |
| Isoflavones/genistein | 100 mg/60 mg, with food |
| B vitamins | A high-dose multiple B-complex, with food |

*Medications*

> Aricept (Donepezil, an "acetylcholine esterase inhibitor" made by Pfizer and Eisa I pharmaceutical companies)
> CDP choline (not yet approved by the FDA)

# CHAPTER 6

# PARKINSON'S DISEASE

No doubt about it: The tremor in his right hand was getting worse. Mark had first noticed it almost a year ago, but because it seemed to happen only after working out at the gym, he attributed the shaking to his advancing years and to his new routine with free weights. After all, he was nearly sixty-eight years old, and how many men his age still exercised regularly?

"No pain, no gain," Mark told himself, and so he kept up his workouts, hoping to improve the muscle fatigue over time.

However, lately he felt tired all the time. His wife was always telling him to speak up, because she could hardly hear him. Another funny thing—and Mark might not have noticed this by itself—was that his skin seemed oilier, almost like when he was in his teens.

Mark, who had celebrated his sixty-fifth birthday and retirement by purchasing the sweet little two-seater car of his dreams, waited another eight months to see his physician.

By then, one of his hands shook so badly he could hardly read the newspaper. His handwriting looked like a spider had run across the page. And he felt irritable and depressed for no reason at all.

"I just want to feel better," he told his doctor. "This is the time in my life when I should really be taking advantage of my freedom and enjoying life. What's wrong with me?"

When his doctor diagnosed Parkinson's disease, Mark felt as if the floor had dropped out from under him. "So what do I do now?" he asked.

## Parkinson's Disease: An Overview

Like most of us, Mark attributed his muscle fatigue and tremor to the normal aging process. However, in Mark's case—as with one out of every forty people—these were early symptoms of Parkinson's disease.

A neurological disease of late middle age, Parkinson's disease affects more than a million Americans. Up to 50,000 new cases are diagnosed each year. Some experts maintain that the disease is increasing in the population and predict it will soon affect one out of every twenty Americans over age fifty.

This slow degenerative nervous disorder most frequently attacks people in their late fifties or sixties. However, more physicians are now reporting cases of Parkinson's in younger patients. Some estimate that up to 10 percent of Parkinson's patients are now diagnosed before they turn forty.

First described in 1817 by James Parkinson, a British physician who published a medical report on "the shaking palsy," Parkinson's disease is characterized by tremor, slowness of movement, and rigidity. Although it is rarely a cause of death, Parkinson's can weaken sufferers enough to fall prey to other diseases.

While researchers have not yet fully defined its causes, range of symptoms, or a cure, we now know that Parkinson's symptoms are clearly linked to the progressive deterioration of dopamine-producing cells in the brain.

Normally, nature creates so many of these neurons that we're able to lose them every day without noticing, as these brain cells disintegrate owing to head injuries, toxins, air pollutants, and aging. In fact, we have to lose over 75 percent of our dopamine neurons before our body shows the telltale symptoms of Parkinson's.

Some people suffering from Parkinson's may end up severely handicapped after a decade or less. Others experience few symptoms even twenty-five years post-diagnosis. Recent popular figures to bring Parkinson's to the public eye include the actress Katharine Hepburn and fighter Muhammad Ali.

Society pays an enormous price for Parkinson's disease. According to the National Parkinson's Foundation, medications cost the average patient upwards of $2,500 annually. When office visits, social security payments, nursing home expenditures, and lost income are totaled for Parkinson's patients, experts estimate that the disease costs the United States more than $5.6 billion a year.

That economic cost pales in comparison to the emotional toll the disease exacts on patients, for who wants to spend their "golden" years trapped in a body that shakes uncontrollably or freezes in place, behind a face devoid of expression owing to inactive muscles?

The good news is this: Advances in treating Parkinson's represent one of the major neurological research success stories of the past decade. It is now hailed as one of the few chronic neurological diseases for which we have found effective treatments.

From the onset of symptoms to diagnosis, from treatment to hope on the horizon, in this chapter we discuss Parkinson's disease in light of what we know about the disease's effects on the brain-immune system connection on its most intricate, biochemical level. At the end of the chapter, you will find an aggressive treatment plan based on the most current information available on medications and nutritional therapies.

## What Goes Wrong in Parkinson's Disease, and Why?

Although no specific genes have been identified for Parkinson's, the disease most likely results from an interaction between genetics and enviroment.

### •A Genetic Predisposition

While there is still more work to do in unraveling the genetic basis for Parkinson's disease, scientists today believe that genetically impaired cellular detoxification mechanisms are the key reason why certain individuals are at risk. When neurons are unable to naturally neutralize environmental toxins, the immune system mounts its forces against those invaders—and may end up killing off the body's own neurons in the process.

## • Exposure to Environmental Toxins

Although all of us are exposed to environmental toxins, current epidemiological studies demonstrate that Parkinson's disease is much more prevalent in areas where individuals are more likely to be exposed to toxins like pesticides, carbon monoxide, carbon disulfide, and other environmental contaminants.

In fact, clinical researchers have identified antibodies specifically targeted to brain cells in the cerebrospinal fluid of Parkinson's patients. When the immune system is activated by a combination of impaired cellular detoxification systems and high exposure to toxins, the result is a cascade of responses that damages neurons in certain areas of the brain—in this case, the neurons responsible for producing dopamine, the neurotransmitter that conveys messages from the brain to control muscle movement and balance.

## • The Death of Dopamine-Producing Neurons at the Hands of MPTP and Other Neurotoxins

Just about sixty years after James Parkinson first linked such symptoms as gait disorder, postural leaning, and tremor as a single chronic disease, Parkinson's patients were treated by medications developed by French neurologist and hypnotist Jean-Martin Charcot. Charcot, known as the "father of clinical neurology," used potions derived from jimsonweed, a North American plant. The herbal remedy brought relief from tremor and rigidity.

During the next century, patients with Parkinson's were treated with extracts from the belladonna plant, a cousin of jimsonweed, and following World War II, with extracts of belladonna-like drugs.

Real progress was finally made in the 1950s, when scientists began experimenting with tranquilizers to control high blood pressure. These investigations yielded new information about neurotransmitters, the chemical substances that transfer information between nerve cells in the brain.

By 1960, University of Vienna scientists had conducted autopsies of the brains of Parkinson's patients and found those brains strikingly short on the dopamine neurotransmitter.

Another piece of the Parkinson's puzzle fell into place in the 1980s, when illicit drug dealers made a designer drug to sell as a synthetic heroin. In an effort to boost their profits and the speed of the manufacturing process, these drug dealers inadvertently created a toxic substance known as MPTP. As reported in *Science* by neurologists at Stanford University School of Medicine, people who took the drug developed symptoms of Parkinson's within a week, puzzling physicians unaccustomed to seeing the disease in young people.

Investigators eventually linked their common use of the MPTP-containing drug to the Parkinson's symptoms. Subsequent studies with laboratory animals have revealed that administering MPTP produces Parkinson's-like symptoms.

As a result, today's researchers believe that Parkinson's disease may be acquired by individuals with a genetic predisposition for the disease if they are exposed to environmental neurotoxins with chemical properties similar to MPTP.

A number of those neurotoxins are found in agricultural pesticides and herbicides commonly used in Western countries, where the prevalence of Parkinson's is highest.

Recall that dopamine is a neurotransmitter that helps activate adrenaline to noradrenaline, thus gearing us up for "fight" or "flight" at times of stress. Dopamine also helps regulate our daily moods—as we explain later in our chapter on depression. More relevant for Parkinson's patients, however, is the fact that dopamine levels are directly related to our ability to move our muscles and keep our balance.

The brain cells that produce dopamine are located deep in the brain stem. Most of these are in an area called the "substantia nigra." The name, which means "black substance" in Latin, describes a darkly pigmented area of the brain which is connected to other parts of the basal ganglia by a network of long, twisting nerve fibers.

Once dopamine is manufactured in the substantia nigra, it travels along those nerve fibers, acting as a messenger for the neurological impulses that help regulate our muscular responses and overall motor functions.

Since discovering the link between Parkinson's and low brain levels of dopamine, scientists in several laboratories have been examining the distribution of dopamine receptors, the chemistry of that particular neurotransmitter, and toxin-induced damage specifically to dopamine-containing neurons.

### • Mitochondrial Damage and Neuron Death

Recently, Japanese investigators who published their findings in a 1995 issue of *Biochimica et Biophysica Acta* have concluded that MPTP selectively destroys neurons in the region of the brain that makes dopamine.

In examining the pathogenesis of Parkinson's on a molecular level, these scientists and others have discovered that the cellular damage may be due to a decrease in the mitochondrial electron transfer—especially in the substantia nigra. This led them to conclude that an energy crisis—literally, the respiratory failure of mitochondria—was responsible for the neuron death.

As you may recall, mitochondria are cellular energy factories often dubbed "the powerhouses of the cell" for the way they function within cells to convert glucose into energy.

In neurons, which require large amounts of protein to perform their functional activities, the mitochondria are small slender rods and spheres located randomly throughout the cell body, but typically near nerve terminals.

Each mitochondria organelle is bounded by two membranes: a smooth outer membrane and an inner membrane, which has numerous infoldings. The matrix, the area enclosed by the inner membrane, is about half protein and contains the mitochondria's DNA, or genetic blueprint.

The mitochondrial inner membrane is where oxidative phosphorylation takes place—the chemical process so fundamental to all aspects of cellular life in organisms that rely on oxygen. That's because the mitochondrial membrane is responsible for moving certain metabolites and mineral ions back and forth between the matrix and the surrounding area.

Now, scientists are finally beginning to grasp just how MPTP, the active toxic agent in that street drug we discussed earlier, damages the cellular mitochondria and produces Parkinson's symptoms, particularly in individuals whose cellular detoxification systems may already be genetically impaired in some way.

## •Nitric Oxide: Good Cop, Bad Cop

Some of the most exciting research in the arena of mitochondrial injury and Parkinson's also throws the spotlight directly on the relationship of dopamine loss to neuronal nitric oxide, a neurotransmitter which also occurs naturally in skeletal muscle and which has attracted the spotlight in recent years for its multiple roles.

Once investigators linked MPTP to clinical, biochemical, and neuropathologic changes similar to those occurring in Parkinson's, subsequent studies led researchers to rapidly conclude that the tragic metabolic changes leading to Parkinson's find center stage in the very mitochondria of those cells.

How? Basically, when MPP, a metabolite of MPTP, collects within the mitochondria of the dopamine-containing neurons, it activates excitatory amino acid receptors, causing the mitochondria of those cells to vacuum up more calcium. This increase in calcium sets off heightened free radical production, activating nitric oxide synthesis within the neurons.

It is this step—the generation of free radical nitric oxide within neurons—that serves as a tragic cellular death sentence. That's because nitric oxide combines with superoxide to form peroxynitrite, the most highly toxic free radical in the body. Peroxynitrite essentially leads to cell death by energy deprivation.

According to Professor P. Jenner, DSc of the Neurodegenerative Disease Research Centre at King's College, London, there is solid evidence for increased lipid peroxidation in the substantia nigra of people with Parkinson's disease. This suggests that free radical production in their bodies is on the rampage. Jenner also concludes that Parkinson's patients have a weakened protective antioxidant defense, and that their bodies' natural repair systems for mending free radical damage are not operating efficiently.

In a 1994 issue of the *Annals of the New York Academy of Science,* other investigators concurred with this finding, correlating oxidative stress and the activation of the nitric oxide pathway in the context of cytokine activation. Thus, as with so many neurological disorders, we find that the breakdown of the body's brain-immune system connection and of the immune system itself play an enormous role in causing the disease.

Not only do the brains of Parkinson's patients show a loss of dopamine-producing neurons, they also demonstrate an increase in the number of macrophages that appear to gulp down degenerating neurons. For the immune system's foot soldier macrophages, nitric oxide serves as a signal to step up superoxide production. This cuts back on essential mitochondrial oxidative phosphorylation and increases the spin-off of toxic free radicals—ultimately leading to oxidative stress and cellular death.

Fortunately, the evidence is so compelling that nitric oxide mediates Parkinson's, we can now make use of medications and nutritional compounds to turn that process around.

In simplest terms, if we can prevent neurons from oversynthesizing nitric oxide in the first place, peroxynitrite won't be around to kill off the brain's dopamine-producing neurons.

Neurologist M. Flint Beal at the Massachusetts General Hospital and his associates in the United States and France have done exactly that. In studies with baboons, they administered MPTP and discovered that the drug produced a dopamine depletion of up to 98 percent in certain parts of the brain, causing the primates to suffer Parkinson's symptoms.

Then, by administering a drug called 7NI (7-nitroindazole), the researchers discovered that they could counter the effect of the neurotoxin by inhibiting nitric acid production, successfully protecting the animals against MPTP-induced dopamine depletion.

## • The Devastating Effects of Lowered Glutathione Levels

One of the body's free radical terminators, glutathione is a naturally occurring amino acid produced in all cells of the body as part of your body's natural detoxification system. Glutathione is particularly effective when it comes to neutralizing free radical attacks on fat.

Because cellular mitochondria churn out so many free radicals in the course of their work on the body's behalf, glutathione deficiency can lead to widespread mitochondrial damage.

Now, scientists have discovered yet another link between lowered glutathione levels and Parkinson's disease. In a study published in 1994 by the *Annals of Neurology,* researchers measured glutathione and oxidized glutathione levels in various areas of the brain in patients dying from Parkinson's. Not surprisingly, these investigators also discovered that the glutathione levels were reduced.

Since glutathione is one of the body's most important naturally occurring antioxidants, this finding is consistent with the concept of oxidative stress as a major component in the death of dopamine-producing neurons.

# A Complete Blueprint for Care

If you or a loved one is diagnosed with Parkinson's disease, the first question to ask is whether Parkinson's is impeding function and quality of life.

If the answer is no, then we recommend avoiding medication until symptoms worsen. In our experience, the longer a patient with Parkinson's is able to get by comfortably without taking medication, the less chance there is of the medication losing efficacy in later stages of the disease.

However, we do believe that patients with Parkinson's should immediately begin a nutritional therapy that combines a low-protein diet with neuroimmunomodulating nutritional substances that have proved to be of benefit in mending the brain-immune connection for people with this disease.

Why this particular protocol? Remember that, with Parkinson's

TABLE **4**

## A CASCADE OF BRAIN CELL DAMAGE

1. Genetic defects impair the natural ability of dopamine-producing brain cells to naturally cleanse themselves of toxins.

2. The susceptible individual is exposed to environmental toxins (pesticides, viruses, heavy metals).

3. There is trauma to the head.

4. The immune system is called into action as a result of 1, 2, 3, or a combination of those factors.

5. Cells are subjected to oxidative stress via free radicals.

6. Cellular mitochondria are damaged and unable to convert energy needed for healthy cellular reactions.

7. Dopamine-producing neurons are damaged or die.

disease, patients may suffer from excessive free radical damage caused by a combination of (1) impaired cellular detoxification systems, (2) exposure to toxins, (3) an immune system gone haywire, and (4) lowered levels of naturally cleansing antioxidants such as glutathione.

Thus, our neuroimmunomodulating therapy for Parkinson's disease consists of boosting the body's own antioxidants through nutritional substances. Additionally, we ask patients to modify their intake of protein, calories, fiber, and fluids to maximize the benefits of therapy while avoiding constipation and dehydration—common complaints of people with Parkinson's.

The earlier this nutritional therapy is begun, the earlier we can help ameliorate or even halt the relentless progress of this disease, as the neuroprotective nutrients we recommend will help preserve the remaining dopamine-producing neurons.

## When Should You Suspect Parkinson's Disease?

Parkinson's disease strikes men and women in almost equal numbers. Early symptoms of the disease are subtle and occur gradually. Not everyone is affected the same way. In some individuals, the disease rampages through the body, causing early disability, while others experience only minor motor disruptions.

Parkinson's may involve one or both sides of the body with anywhere from mild postural imbalance to critical instability. Patients afflicted with severe Parkinson's may eventually be restricted to a bed or chair. Some patients indicate that their early symptoms appeared during periods of stress, then subsided, only to reappear several years later on a more consistent basis.

Tremor is the major symptom for some Parkinson's patients, while for others tremor is only a minor complaint and different symptoms pose more problems. The tremor associated with Parkinson's takes on a characteristic appearance that physicians call "pill rolling."

Typically, tremor begins in a hand, and takes the form of a rhythmic back-and-forth motion of forefinger and thumb. It is most obvious when someone is under stress. Tremor may also affect a foot or jaw first. In most patients, the tremor affects only one side or one part of the body during early stages of the disease.

The second symptom common to most Parkinson's patients is rigidity, or resistance to movement. A major principle of body movement is that all muscles have an opposing muscle. In other words, you are able to move a muscle not just because it becomes more active, but because the opposing muscle relaxes.

Parkinson's patients experience rigidity because communication between the brain and the muscles is disturbed. Instead of relaxing, the opposing muscles remain constantly tensed to the point of aching. The rigidity becomes obvious when another person tries to move the patient's arm and is able to do so only in jerky, ratchetlike movements.

The third symptom, bradykinesia, is often the most frustrating. The term describes the slowing down of spontaneous and automatic muscle movement—like the movements you use to wash or dress—so that common daily activities take hours instead of minutes.

In the advanced stages of Parkinson's, patients experience postural instability which may cause them to lean and fall over easily. As the disease progresses, Parkinson's patients may halt in mid-stride and "freeze" in place, possibly even tipping over. Or they may walk with quick, tiny steps to keep their balance as they move forward.

Various other symptoms may accompany Parkinson's as well, such as depression and emotional changes. Many patients lose their motivation and become dependent on family members. About a third of Parkinson's patients also suffer memory loss.

## Diagnosing Parkinson's: A Complex Masquerade

One of the difficulties in finding ways to inhibit or reverse the neurological deterioration in Parkinson's disease is the long delay in diagnosis. Too often, patients are not diagnosed until full-blown symptoms develop—which means they have already experienced at least a 70–80 percent decrease in the neurons we rely on to make dopamine, the neurotransmitter so essential for muscle control. To effectively treat Parkinson's patients, an early diagnosis is imperative.

However, even for an experienced neurologist, it is sometimes difficult to make an accurate diagnosis in the early stages of Parkinson's, as there is no sophisticated blood or laboratory test available to date.

Complicating things further is the fact that Parkinson's can masquerade as other conditions, including:

- Neurological disorders resulting from stroke, tumors, and head traumas
- Metabolic conditions, such as hypoparathyroidism
- Symptoms brought on by major tranquilizers and antinausea drugs
- Benign essential tremor

To ensure a correct early diagnosis of Parkinson's, the physician may need to observe you or your loved one for some time, until it is apparent that a tremor is present and one or more of the other classic symptoms are also manifest. Another potentially promising laboratory marker for the diagnosis of Parkinson's disease involves measuring the amount of free radical activity in white blood cells, which appears higher than normal in Parkinson's patients.

## The First Step to Take: Begin a Low-Protein Diet

It is sometimes difficult for investigators to determine the effects of disease progression in Parkinson's patients, because there are some patients with Parkinson's who reveal only one or two symptoms for many years, while others worsen rapidly after diagnosis. However, there is a solid, scientific foundation for using a low-protein diet and taking the neuroimmunomodulating nutritional supplements we recommend below as a means of preserving the remaining healthy dopamine-producing neurons.

Because the human body converts protein to amino acids, a low-protein diet may help Parkinson's patients by allowing more dopamine to become available in the brain.

This is a simple matter of competition: the precursors of dopamine include the amino acid tyrosine, which is converted in the body in a series of steps first to dopa and then to dopamine. Dopa ends up competing with other amino acids to enter through the blood-brain barrier. If fewer amino acids are available, then more dopa can be rushed past the border guards and into the brain, where it can be converted to dopamine.

In addition, some researchers have found that high protein diets may actually increase the risk of dying from Parkinson's disease. For example, physicians at Georgetown University's School of Medicine have conducted comparative studies of Parkinson's patients in countries as diverse as the United States, Mexico, and Japan. They found a striking correlation between high levels of dietary protein and death from Parkinson's. Low-protein diets therefore may offer more than just symptomatic relief to Parkinson's patients.

In summary, then, because the large, neutral amino acids derived from dietary proteins compete with dopa—an essential natural precursor to dopamine synthesis—we recommend that patients take just 10 percent of their allotted daily protein during the day, with the bulk of dietary protein to be consumed at night. That allows dopa to make its way to the brain with as little competition from other amino acids as possible. Studies have demonstrated that patients who restrict their protein intake to the evening meal show greater improvement than those who do not.

It's important to note, in adjusting the diet to better manage Parkinson's, that many patients with the disease are at risk for malnutrition owing to a variety of factors, including low income, social isolation, impaired appetite, depression, dementia, inactivity, and increased metabolic requirements.

Therefore, in addition to restricting protein intake, we urge Parkinson's patients to maintain an ideal body weight through adequate caloric intake (between 12 and 16 calories per pound of body weight).

## Other Dietary Suggestions for Managing Parkinson's

### • Enhance Fluid and Fiber Intake

Studies have demonstrated that a diet rich in insoluble fiber lessens constipation while increasing the availability of dopa for uptake by the brain's neurons.

We suggest incorporating insoluble types of fiber into your diet throughout the day through foods such as wheat bran, rice bran, whole wheat breads, crackers, and cereals. In addition, we ask patients to drink a minimum of eight glasses of water daily to avoid constipation. Another route we recommend is to take miller's bran and psyllium fiber supplements as directed by your nutritionist or physician. Lastly, the use of "friendly" bacteria is crucial in maintaining normal bowel flora and regulation. Look for a combination product that contains both lactobaccilli and bifido organisms.

### •Ensure Adequate Antioxidant Foods

The hallmark of Parkinson's disease is a lowered level of gluta-thione, the detoxifying free radical scavenger that is especially important to protecting brain cells. Our neuroprotective therapy is based on boosting deficiencies in antioxidants and important antioxidant enzyme systems such as glutathione peroxidase.

Patients with insufficient intake of antioxidants such as vita-mins C and E, tocotrienols, selenium, carotenoids, N-acetyl-cysteine, and glutathione run the risk of free radicals rampaging through the body and causing further damage to already weak-ened cells.

Dr. Stanley Fahn, a professor of neurology at Columbia Presby-terian Hospital and a world-renowned researcher in Parkinson's disease, has presented a considerable body of evidence in both human and animal models to support the concept of oxidative stress heightening the pathology of Parkinson's.

Among the evidence supporting this concept is the fact that the brains of patients with Parkinson's have increased lipid perox-idation, reduced levels of glutathione, increased iron, and by-products of oxidant stress, such as abnormal enzyme activity. As a result of this evidence, clinicians are now recommending that patients with Parkinson's receive aggressive antioxidant treat-ment.

### •Avoid Certain Supplements

In a 1995 issue of *Toxicology,* University of Arizona College of Medicine researcher Dr. Erwin Montgomery reviewed the role of heavy metals such as iron and manganese in Parkinson's disease. According to his report, the combination of high iron and the nerve transmitter dopamine may result in free radical damage to the brain's substantia nigra. Also, dopamine may break down and produce free radicals in the presence of iron and other heavy metals, such as manganese and copper.

A number of other investigators concur with this finding, while still others have ferreted out evidence of elevated iron levels and enhanced oxidative damage in the substantia nigra of Parkinson's disease patients.

Based on these and other findings, we recommend that patients with Parkinson's should not only step up their intake of antioxidants, but also steer away from supplements of iron, manganese, and choline—all of which have been shown to worsen the progression of Parkinson's or to be correlated with developing the disease in the first place.

### •*Add Beans as a Natural Dopa Source*

Consider using broad beans, such as faba beans (also known as fava), in place of protein during the day. While most broad beans are a good source of naturally occurring dopa, researchers reporting in *Nutrition Reviews* have found that the vicia faba bean is a particularly rich source and may have some use in managing Parkinson motor fluctuations. Additionally, faba beans are high in fiber and contain dopa in a form different from that found in prescription medication. Just one 3.5-ounce serving of vicia faba beans contains 250 mg of dopa in its free form.

## Nutritional Supplements You Should Begin Incorporating Now

### • *NADH (Nicotinamide Adenine Dinucleotide): An Early Stop on the Dopamine Assembly Line*

In the brain's assembly line for producing the essential dopamine neurotransmitter, one of the earliest stops is with an enzyme called tyrosine hydroxylase, which helps convert the amino acid tyrosine to dopa, dopamine's precursor. This reaction requires a substance called BH4, a compound produced in the brain with the help of NADH.

In studies by Dr. George Birkmayer of the Birkmayer Institute for Parkinson's Therapy in Vienna, Austria, Parkinson's patients taking NADH significantly improved their ability to walk, push, stand upright, and speak when treated with NADH. Upon withdrawing NADH, disabling symptoms of the disease returned within three weeks.

Birkmayer's research is supported by other studies showing that the level of BH4 is cut in half in the brains of Parkinson's patients, and by tissue culture research showing that NADH does indeed increase tyrosine hydroxylase activity and dopamine production.

NADH is a safe, natural compound that you can purchase over the counter at any health food store. It will come under further scrutiny in the decade to come. Meanwhile, we recommend supplementation with NADH as part of the nutrition protocol for Parkinson's patients, as a way of assisting with the production of BH4 and subsequently activating the brain's natural production of L-Dopa and dopamine.

RECOMMENDED DOSE:   10 mg daily, divided into two 5 mg doses.

## •Antioxidants

When the body's immune system mobilizes, our cells use more oxygen and consequently produce by-products called oxygen free radicals. These free radicals destroy invaders efficiently by attacking their very biological components and mechanisms. Unfortunately, they can also terrorize our own cells, chewing through cellular membranes in their search for electrons to steal and even dismantling the very DNA that contains cellular genetic codes.

In Parkinson's, we know that the neurotransmitter nitric oxide penetrates dopamine-producing neurons and combines with superoxide to form peroxynitrite, the most highly toxic free radical in the body. Peroxynitrite essentially leads to cell death by energy deprivation.

Studies have shown that Parkinson's disease is exacerbated by a chronic antioxidant deficiency state. As we previously discussed, drug therapy for Parkinson's may also add to the free radical damage to neurons.

A large study conducted in the 1980s looked at the effect of using vitamin E as a therapeutic agent in treating Parkinson's and found that vitamin E had little or no effect on the rate of disease progression. However, we now know that antioxidants work more effectively in concert with one another than in isolation. This is because each antioxidant performs differently in the body. Clinical nutrition is not practiced using the "single magic bullet" approach, but rather with the recognition that a synergistic array of nutrients represents a more efficient approach.

So, while taking a single antioxidant may not impede Parkinson's, we recommend that all patients with Parkinson's take a complete antioxidant supplement and add additional amounts of the glutathione-boosting antioxidants, lipoic acid, NAC, and selenium.

Below, we discuss the role of iron in oxidative damage to the brain's substantia nigra—the region where most of our brain dopamine is produced—as well as the antioxidants essential in a nutritional protocol specific to treating Parkinson's disease.

RECOMMENDED DOSE: In addition to the therapeutic dosages of specific antioxidants suggested below for people who have been diagnosed with Parkinson's, we urge all Parkinson's patients to add a complete advanced antioxidant formula, takine in the amounts prescribed on the label.

### • Lipoic Acid: Add This to Your First Line of Defense

Along with vitamins E and C, lipoic acid is probably the most important antioxidant in the first line of defense against free radical damage for Parkinson's patients. Unlike vitamin C, which is water soluble, and vitamin E, which is fat soluble, lipoic acid has the capability to act as a freee radical scavenger in both the body's fat cell compartments and the water cell compartments.

Lipoic acid is environmentally conscious, and recycles other important antioxidants, including C, E, and coenzyme Q10. Lipoic acid and n-acetyl-cysteine (NAC) can raise the body's glutathione production as well—an essential feature for Parkinson's patients, since they have reduced levels of glutathione. Additionally, the mineral selenium is essential as a component of glutathione antioxidant enzymes.

What is glutathione, and why is it so important to support its production by taking lipoic acid supplements? An amino acid that occurs naturally in our diets and is produced by healthy cells as part of the body's housekeeping system, glutathione protects every organ, tissue, and cell in the body against free radical damage. Various studies have shown that people with high levels of glutathione have more efficient immune activity.

Because studies show that blood levels of glutathione drop drastically as we age, and because Parkinson's patients have impaired antioxidant defense systems, we recommend that people with Parkinson's disease supplement the glutathione they get in their diets through food. The best sources of glutathione include acorn squash, asparagus, avocado, grapefruit, oranges, potatoes, strawberries, tomatoes, watermelon, cauliflower, broccoli, and cantaloupe.

As we explained earlier, because taking glutathione orally is ineffective because the body cannot efficiently absorb it, it is far more efficient to boost the body's glutathione levels by taking supplements of NAC (n-acetyl-cysteine), lipoic acid, and selenium to increase the body's natural glutathione synthesis.

**RECOMMENDED DAILY DOSES:**

| | |
|---|---|
| Lipoic acid | 200 mg, with a meal |
| NAC (n-acetyl-cysteine) | 1 g, on an empty stomach |
| Selenium | 200 mcg, with a meal (Do not exceed this dose.) |

## •Tocopherols and Tocotrienols: Powerful Antioxidant Allies

Tocopherols (Vitamin E) and tocotrienols are major lipid-soluble antioxidants that protect our bodies against free radical damage. Tocotrienols are less widely distributed in nature than tocopherols, and are slightly different in chemical structure, allowing them to penetrate fatty tissue more efficiently. This is particularly important in treating Parkinson's, as the brain is mostly fatty tissue.

While tocopherols are readily available in corn, soybean, olive, and other vegetable oils, you need to turn to rice, bran, and barley oils to find tocotrienols. We recommend a combination of both kinds of oils to offer the best protection against lipid oxidation in the body.

RECOMMENDED DOSES: Up to 800 IUs of tocopherols and 60 mg of tocotrienols each day.

## • Coenzyme Q10: The Energetic Antioxidant

As a lipid-soluble compound found in mitochondria, coenzyme Q10 plays a major role in energy production. Since free radical mitochondria damage results in altered electron transport and cellular death owing to energy deficiency, supplemental coenzyme Q10 may be especially beneficial in treating Parkinson's.

A study by Harvard Medical School researcher J. B. Shultz and his colleagues, published in a 1995 issue of *Experimental Neurology*, revealed that coenzyme Q10 protects against MPTP, the neurotoxin we discussed earlier that produces the symptoms of Parkinson's and causes the death and destruction of essential dopamine-producing neurons.

Additional studies demonstrate that coenzyme Q10 provides better protection against the oxidation of fats than vitamin E. Some investigators conclude that this antioxidant may actually go beyond just protecting membrane lipids to defend proteins and DNA against oxidative damage.

RECOMMENDED DOSE: 200 mg daily, with a meal.

## • Polyphenols: The Colorful Antioxidants

Polyphenols are a large class of compounds that encompass both bioflavonoids and proanthocyanidins. These are the pigment materials responsible for the richly varied scents, tastes, and coloring of many fruits and plants.

Most significantly, proanthocyanidins are renowned for their superior antioxidant properties and efficient bioavailability— that is, better absorption and utilization. In fact, a number of nutritional scientists describe them as the most powerful naturally occurring free radicals to date.

One important attribute shared by proanthocyanidins is that, unlike other bioflavonoids, they are allowed past the border guards of the blood-brain barrier and can permeate that chemical "wall" freely. While no present studies indicate the effect of proanthocyanidins in treating Parkinson's, we recommend including them in this nutritional protocol based on their superb antioxidant properties.

> RECOMMENDED DOSE: 120 mg of a polyphenol supplement, daily, such as Pycnogenol®, green tea, grape seed, or fruit polyphenols, taken with a meal.

## Detoxification Supplements: Assisting the Liver in Cleansing the Body's Tissues

As we discussed earlier in this chapter, neurotoxins from both internal and external environments most likely play a role in causing Parkinson's disease. Several studies have demonstrated that Parkinson's patients have abnormal liver enzymes that may hamper the ability of the liver to cleanse the body's tissues of toxins.

For example, in an article published in *Geriatrics,* Dr. Caroline M. Tanner reviewed the possibilities of abnormal liver enzymes as contributors to Parkinson's and suggested that vulnerability to toxins among Parkinson's patients may be due, in part, to impaired liver enzymes. Researching the role of hepatic enzymes in Parkinson's may very well be the first crucial step in discovering more intervention and preventive therapies for treating the disease.

Further studies will determine just which hepatic enzymes are involved. Meanwhile, we strongly encourage people with Parkinson's to add a regimen of liver support agents. These nutritional supplements have the potential to enhance the ability of the liver to conduct its detoxifying duties more rigorously.

> RECOMMENDED DOSES: We recommend adding 300 mg daily of standardized milk thistle herb as a liver support

nutrient. The lipoic acid and NAC discussed earlier are also important for liver function.

## What Other Medical Therapies Should You Discuss with Your Health Care Provider?

If the symptoms of Parkinson's worsen to the point that they impair function and cause a decline in quality of life, we suggest that patients with Parkinson's discuss the possibility of combining medication with nutritional substances in this neuroimmunomodulating therapy.

***Sinemet.*** Sinemet, a drug that combines L-Dopa with carbidopa, is unquestionably the best symptomatic treatment for Parkinson's today. However, as some studies show that treatment with L-Dopa hastens the appearance of adverse side effects and eventually results in an intolerance of this drug, we recommend treating Parkinson's symptoms with this agent only when the disease is causing a functional disability based on the patient's individual needs. Common side effects include nausea, vomiting, and sometimes hallucinations.

***Pergolide or Permax.*** An "agonist" is a chemical with the ability to work together with a neurotransmitter and enhance its action. Pergolide or Permax is a dopamine agonist proved to be beneficial in slowing the rate of Parkinson's and in treating symptoms.

In a seven-year follow-up study conducted with Parkinson's patients who took pergolide, for example, researchers in Rochester, New York, discovered that the subgroup of participants who received pergolide for up to seven years showed an absence of clinical progression of Parkinson's. In related studies, investigators have found that chronic pergolide administered to rats slowed the age-related loss of dopamine-containing neurons.

***Deprenyl.*** A number of studies have shown that Deprenyl can decrease the symptoms of Parkinson's in some patients by blocking the enzyme that controls how much dopamine is broken down.

By putting the brakes on this enzyme, called monoamine

oxidase B, dopamine supplies are allowed to build up again in the brain. A multicenter study reported in the *New England Journal of Medicine* showed that Deprenyl slowed the progress of Parkinson's disease and delayed the need for symptomatic treatment with Sinemet until later.

## Putting It All Together

For more than two years now, Mark has maintained his health by switching to a low-protein diet, stepping up his intake of antioxidant- and fiber-rich foods, and adding a general antioxidant supplement as well as 200 mg of lipoic acid, 1.5 g of NAC, 120 mg of coenzyme Q10, and 300 mg of standardized milk thistle extract to boost his cellular glutathione production and strengthen his liver's detoxification function. As a preventive measure, we put Mark on Deprenyl as well.

This combination of mediating his diet and increasing his intake of antioxidants, along with taking Deprenyl to block the enzyme that controls how much dopamine is broken down, has seemed to stabilize Mark's symptoms for the time being, thus delaying the need to treat Mark with a symptomatic therapy such as Sinemet.

In addition, we have encouraged Mark to work with an experienced physical therapist in a movement therapy program designed to help him maintain and strengthen his motor activity. Performing a series of physical therapy exercises each day helps Mark strengthen his muscles and maintain coordination.

Happily, Mark has continued to function well on his own for these two years since diagnosis without the need of a home health aide or any additional care by his wife. In fact, a recent exam showed that Mark has not experienced any further neurological deterioration.

Now that you have an overview of Parkinson's disease and how it affects the very structure, function, and biochemical metabolism of the brain–immune system connection, you are probably eager to get started—or to help someone you love begin—investigating a complete treatment protocol.

For all patients with Parkinson's disease, we recommend a

low-protein diet rich in antioxidant foods. In addition, here is our summary guideline for treatment.

*Daily Nutritional Supplements*

| | |
|---|---|
| Antioxidants | A complete antioxidant supplement, taken in the amounts prescribed by the formula label. The formula should include a full carotenoid complex containing alpha and beta carotene totaling up to 25,000 IU, with lutein and lycopene. |
| Vitamin E | Up to 800 IU alpha and mixed tocopherols and up to 60 mg tocotrienols. |
| Selenium | 200 mcg, with food |
| Lipoic acid | 200 mg, with food |
| NAC (n-acetyl-cysteine) | 1 g, on an empty stomach |
| Coenzyme Q10 | 200 mg, with food |
| Standardized milk thistle | 300 mg, with food |
| Polyphenols | 120 mg, of a polyphenol supplement such as green tea, grape seed extract, Pycogenol®, or fruit polyphenols |

If constipation is present, patients should add a multiple-strain "friendly bacteria" product between meals, increase fluid intake, and possibly add miller's bran or psyllium seed husks to the diet as described in our chapter on gut-supporting nutrients.

*Protective Medications (to prevent progression)*

Deprenyl
Pergolide (Permax)

*Symptomatic Therapies*

Sinemet

# MULTIPLE SCLEROSIS

Regina was just twenty-eight years old when she first started experiencing numbness and tingling in her left foot. She ignored the sensation, since it wasn't painful, and soon enough the symptoms went away.

It was during her divorce nearly two years later, after a bad bout with the flu, that the numbness returned. However, this time she felt the strange feeling in both feet. She was anxious these days, and having a lot of trouble sleeping, but she attributed all her symptoms to the increased stress in her life. After all, here she was, suddenly a single mother of two young children and working full-time besides.

Her doctor found nothing wrong and prescribed antidepressants. The symptoms receded, and she didn't think much more about them—other than to be thankful that she was feeling good again. Then, just a year later, she suddenly lost the vision in one eye while reading the newspaper.

That's when her family doctor sent Regina to a neurologist. An MRI scan of her brain revealed the classic plaques of multiple sclerosis on the nerve fibers in her brain, confirming the neurologist's suspicions.

# Multiple Sclerosis: An Overview

In recent decades, investigators have been relentless in their search for understanding the causes of multiple sclerosis and the development of new treatment protocols aimed at throwing a stumbling block in its path. They have succeeded in ferreting out a great deal of information. Yet, many practitioners still catalogue multiple sclerosis as a chronic disease for which there is no known cause or cure.

In fact, multiple sclerosis affects about 300,000 Americans in ways as various as the individuals whose lives it strikes. For some, the disease is relatively mild. Others experience severe disability. Although there are no magic bullets for curing multiple sclerosis, it is now possible to aggressively—and successfully—treat the disease.

Multiple sclerosis typically affects women of childbearing age and almost always strikes adults between the ages of thirty and fifty. The term "multiple sclerosis" literally means "many scars," and refers to the scarring on the nerve fibers—or plaques—caused by the disease.

The plaques, which are readily seen with today's MRI techniques, represent areas on nerve cell fibers in the brain and spinal cord where the myelin—the fatty insulation covering the fibers—has worn away. These gaps in myelin sheathing interfere with the high-speed transmission of electrical messages between the central nervous system and the rest of the body.

Although multiple sclerosis is categorized as a neurological disease, it is also a disease of the immune system. For patients with multiple sclerosis, the immune system turns against the body instead of defending it—thus putting multiple sclerosis in the broader category of autoimmune diseases. In other words, multiple sclerosis is a good example of the interrelatedness of our body systems.

In the case of multiple sclerosis, myelin is clearly the target of the immune system's attack. More specifically, the bull's-eye of the target is a myelin basic protein.

You'll read about myelin basic protein later in this chapter. We will also discuss the controversial link between certain dietary fats and multiple sclerosis, and point out the value of nutritional supplements in preventing myelin degeneration.

From the onset of symptoms to diagnosis, from treatment to hope on the horizon, in this chapter we discuss multiple sclerosis in the light of what we know about how the disease affects the brain-immune system on its most intricate biochemical level. At the end of the chapter, you will find an aggressive treatment plan based on the most current information available on medications and nutritional therapies.

## What Goes Wrong in Multiple Sclerosis, and Why?

In multiple sclerosis, normal immunological reactions become damaging because immune cells target the body's own cellular structures—in other words, the immune system loses its capacity to recognize its own body. Our new grasp of what makes otherwise protective immune mechanisms tailspin out of control is the basis for treating the disease today.

As we know, the immune system is normally capable of identifying invaders such as viruses and bacteria by "reading" molecular codes found on cell surfaces. These molecular codes are like the flags of different armies. The immune system will not attack an invader if it sees a flag belonging to its own army.

However, various types of viruses and bacteria successfully camouflage themselves against attack by the immune system with molecular codes on their cell surfaces identical to the components in your own body. Several viruses can play hide-and-seek with the immune system by changing their flag colors to look like the colors sported by its host. These foxy viruses include measles, herpes simplex VI, and the Epstein-Barr virus.

When this happens, the immune system becomes confused and may either ignore the invader completely or go on the offensive against parts of itself. This "molecular mimicry" is especially relevant to multiple sclerosis. Although the mechanism is still not completely understood, scientists now believe that previous exposure to one of these mimicking viruses causes the immune system to create antibodies to that virus. When the virus is no longer around, something prompts the immune system to create antibodies to the body's own brain myelin—which has molecular components bearing an uncanny resemblance to that virus.

Myelin is the fatty insulating substance surrounding nerve sheaths in the brain and spinal cord much the same way we coat electrical wires with protective rubber to ensure effective transmissions. Made up of fats, it is white in appearance and serves to conduct nerve impulses between various regions of the nervous system.

Disruption of myelin, or demyelination, impairs the ability of nerve fibers to transmit impulses and is responsible for many symptoms of multiple sclerosis, including weakness, sensory loss, and visual disturbances. How severely multiple sclerosis affects patients may be directly related to the profusion and locations of the scarring, or plaques, on the brain and spinal cord.

In multiple sclerosis patients, all of the immune system's components are involved in one way or another in this inadvertent attack on the brain's myelin. These components include B cells, T cells, macrophages, and all of the associated cytokines, the chemical mediators serving in this biological warfare.

B cells, as you may recall, are the immune system components responsible for manufacturing immunoglobulins such as IgG, large protein molecules designed to specifically recognize and bind to invading substances—also called the "antigens"—in order to transform them into targets for future attack by other immune system warriors, including T Cells and macrophages.

People with multiple sclerosis have elevated levels of the IgG immunoglobulin in their cerebrospinal fluid, as well as in the brain. Tragically, these IgG protein molecules have chosen to target the myelin basic protein.

Why does this happen? To put it in simplest terms, myelin is made up of lipids, complex fats, and proteins. The immune system can misidentify the myelin basic protein as a foreign substance because it has a similar molecular code as a virus that the multiple sclerosis patient was exposed to earlier in life, such as measles.

Once the B cells go on the attack, warrior T cells and foot soldier macrophages are automatically called into action, further damaging the wrongly victimized brain tissue. T cells perpetuate the biological error, signaling further reserves when they release their cytokines, the chemical mediators of the immune system.

Many studies reveal a clear association between one particular cytokine, called tumor necrosis factor (TNF), and multiple sclerosis attacks. In a two-year study conducted with multiple sclerosis patients between twenty and fifty years old, Dr. Romain Hentges and his colleagues measured the levels of TNF in the cerebrospinal fluid and serum and correlated those levels with the way the disease progressed in each patient.

Their results, which they published in the *New England Journal of Medicine*, demonstrated that over half of the patients with chronic progressive multiple sclerosis had elevated TNF levels. Not one of the patients with stable multiple sclerosis had the same escalating levels of this busy cytokine.

Why would patients with elevated TNF levels suffer more from multiple sclerosis attacks?

When your immune system is working properly, the body's own blood-brain barrier—the cellular and chemical guards that select which substances are granted permission to pass into the brain from the blood capillaries—keeps out invaders.

However, one function of the TNF cytokine is to create passages for other components of the immune system to cross the blood-brain barrier and enter into the battle zone, much the way army engineers build roads and bridges to allow further reserve troops to enter a war zone.

Without the help of TNF, the hand-to-hand combatants of our immune system—our macrophages—could never make it into the front line trenches of the brain. This breakdown of the blood-brain barrier is the first rung on the ladder to multiple sclerosis attacks, for it is followed by inflammation, the breakdown of myelin, and the formation of hard fibrous material (the scars, or sclerosis) on the nerve fibers.

How do the macrophages carry out their assault once they successfully cross the blood-brain barrier? Recall that macrophages are mobile white blood cells which can literally chew off pieces of invaders and engulf them. They damage the brain's myelin by secreting enzymes that break down the molecular components of the sheathing.

The macrophage-produced agents include arachidonic acid,

free radicals, and other inflammatory substances which cause most of the damage to myelin in the immune system attacks common to multiple sclerosis. Gamma interferon, typically produced as a result of viral infections or nonspecific inflammation, joins in to amplify the immune response against myelin.

## Why Does Multiple Sclerosis Affect More Women Than Men?

The estrogen hormone appears to play a role in a number of autoimmune diseases. This is supported by the fact that all autoimmune diseases are far more common in women than in men, particularly during childbearing years when estrogen levels are greatest.

At least part of the reason is that estrogen plays a role in autoimmune diseases is because estrogen stimulates the production of gamma interferon in the immune system. Gamma interferon, which is also found in the ovaries and may be manufactured there as well as in the immune system, activates macrophages and enhances the ability of T cells to target foreign substances—immune responses which are particularly detrimental in multiple sclerosis.

## Why Are Multiple Sclerosis Attacks Often Linked to Stress?

Stress is interpreted by the body as a danger signal and results in the "fight or flight" response which affects both the brain and the immune system. On a biochemical level, the fight or flight system involves the brain's production of hormones and their influence on the adrenal glands and immune cells. This triad is known as the brain-adrenal-immune axis.

Today, we know that the brain regions involved in the fight or flight response include the hypothalamus, which releases corticotropin-releasing factor (CRF) and the pituitary, which releases ACTH. These two hormones directly influence the adrenal glands to increase the manufacture and release of cortisol, which in turn allows the muscles, brain, and heart to metabolize more glucose and have the energy at hand to respond to threatening events.

According to researchers at the National Institute of Mental Health, immune cytokines not only activate immune function when you're under stress, they also recruit the neurotransmitters essential in modulating your immune response and activating behaviors that may be important during injury or inflammation.

These investigators suggest that diseases characterized by both inflammation and emotional stress—like multiple sclerosis—may be the result of common alterations in the brain–immune system connection. Cytokines produced by immune-inflammatory cells such as interleukin and TNF (tumor necrosis factor) stimulate parts of the brain, including the hypothalamus, to secrete corticotropin-releasing hormone and cause a chemical domino effect. The last domino down is the release of corticosteroids.

Corticosteroids function to suppress inflammation and the immune response. To understand why your body's primary response to stress, in essence, is to produce larger amounts of cortisol, think of it this way: The effect of heightened cortisol production is to suppress the immune system's responses. And that's only logical, for why should your body care about fighting an infection when you need extra energy to combat a more immediate danger?

This suppressive effect is typically short-lived. Once the immediate danger is removed, your immune system should recover. In other words, during periods of acute stress, your body produces heightened levels of cortisol and a decrease in inflammation.

However, during periods of chronic stress, this sustained increase in cortisol is capable of derailing the immune system in ways that persist far beyond immediate goals. This derailment is analogous to "the boy who cried wolf," in that the danger signals are ignored because of their persistence. The inflammation continues, because the cortisol receptors have blunted the immunosuppressant response.

Clinicians typically define stress as life events that require significant changes in behavior to readjust to them. Since research into a possible relationship between stress and illness began half a century ago, a number of studies have linked emotional stress to illnesses as varied as tuberculosis, ulcers, heart attacks, leukemia, juvenile diabetes, and a general susceptibility to illness. Now researchers believe that stress can be one of the components of any disease.

In patients with multiple sclerosis, stress unleashes destructive immune processes from their normal regulatory constraints. As we saw in Regina's case, a multiple sclerosis attack is often preceded by a stressful life event such as a divorce. A number of researchers have examined the lives of multiple sclerosis patients and discovered relationships between the disease and emotional stress.

## Infections: Another Kind of Stress

As we saw in Chapter 1, infections provoke the immune system into action. Common viral, urinary tract, and yeast infections can all prod the immune system and result in a relapse for multiple sclerosis patients when the foreign invader produces a state of heightened alertness by the immune system.

# A Complete Blueprint for Care

In the section below, we outline a complete blueprint for care of patients with multiple sclerosis. This plan combines the latest information on the benefits of low-fat diets and neuroimmuno-modulating substances you can add to your diet right away.

Perhaps more than any other neurological illness described in these pages, the severity of multiple sclerosis attacks has been clearly linked to stress. Therefore, all patients diagnosed with multiple sclerosis should consider including such support as psychotherapy or counseling groups, meditation, and biofeedback as a first step toward treating the disease.

In addition to modulating stress, multiple sclerosis patients can immediately begin decreasing the number of pro-inflammatory immune cells and increasing anti-inflammatory immune cells by adopting a low-fat diet and adding nutritional supplements

### TABLE 5

## MULTIPLE SCLEROSIS: A CASCADE OF MYELIN DAMAGE

1. The body is exposed early to a virus which mimics myelin basic protein, such as herpes simplex VI, Epstein-Barr virus, adenovirus, or measles.
2. The immune system calls B cells into action, making IgG.
3. IgG binds to myelin basic protein, further identifying it as a foreign invader.
4. T cells respond to the IgG signal, starting the next phase of immune response: the production of tumor necrosis factor and gamma interferon cytokines.
5. Tumor necrosis factor paves the way for macrophages to begin devouring "invaders."
6. Macrophages use toxic biological weaponry, such as arachidonic acid and free radicals, to chew off neuron myelin and impair electrical transmission between the central nervous system and muscles.

that are readily available at your health food store. These neuroimmunomodulating agents include PS (phosphatidylserine) and antioxidants.

## When Should You Suspect Multiple Sclerosis?

There are three types of multiple sclerosis. The first, and most common, is the "relapse-remitting" form of the disease, where an attack with full-blown symptoms is followed by a period of remission when the body returns to its former state or to a slightly worsened state.

In some individuals, however, the disease can take a more chronic, progressive path with very few instances of remission. Rarer still is the case of "galloping" multiple sclerosis, where the disease moves quickly through the body and causes rapid debilitation.

Early signs of multiple sclerosis include the following:

- A tingling sensation in the extremities
- Dragging either foot while walking
- Loss of sensation and coordination
- Blurred or double vision
- Problems urinating
- Abnormal fatigue, to the point where even common daily activities are too tiring

## Diagnosing Multiple Sclerosis

Over the past decade, physicians have armed themselves with a number of tests to diagnose multiple sclerosis. Early tests involved drawing blood samples and analyzing it for the presence of abnormal amounts of IgG or red cell mobility. Today's neurologists rely on CAT (computed axial tomography) scans, MRI (magnetic resonance imaging), and analysis of immunological markers in cerebrospinal fluid. These scanning devices all help pinpoint specific tissue damage such as plaques, atrophy, and inflammation.

Multiple sclerosis symptoms mimic those of other disorders, including Lyme disease, certain viral infections, other autoimmune diseases such as lupus, and B12 deficiency. It is essential to rule these disorders out during diagnosis, as many of them are easily treatable.

### •*Lyme Disease*

Endemic to certain areas of the United States, Lyme disease is spread by ticks. It may be characterized by a bull's-eye-shaped rash, fever, and swollen, painful joints. However, these symptoms are not inevitable, and Lyme disease may produce a clinical state that is very similar to multiple sclerosis, including demyelination of the brain. Unfortunately, the routine blood test for Lyme disease may not be specific or sensitive enough to give an accurate result. To adequately determine whether the symptoms are caused by Lyme or multiple sclerosis, the physician may order a spinal tap with analysis of Lyme in the cerebrospinal fluid.

### • Lupus, Sjogren's Syndrome and Other Autoimmune Diseases

All autoimmune diseases require blood testing to determine the presence of certain antibodies that serve as biological markers.

### • B12 Deficiency

A deficiency of the B12 vitamin can cause demyelination, as normal B12 levels are required for adequate myelin synthesis. Patients with multiple sclerosis should be screened for B12 deficiency, as such a deficiency requires treatment.

## Dietary Suggestions for Patients with Multiple Sclerosis

### • Begin a Low-Fat Diet

As in the case of so many other chronic diseases, saturated fats do terrible damage to blood vessel walls in multiple sclerosis patients. A diet high in saturated fats causes platelets in the blood to bunch together and stretch blood vessel walls. When the blood-brain barrier breaks down, toxic materials seep through the blood into the brain and a cascade of immune responses begins, resulting in the myelin breakdown and scarring of nerve fibers so characteristic of multiple sclerosis.

Investigators now believe that a diet low in saturated fat is one of the best tools in the fight against multiple sclerosis. Shifting to certain polyunsaturated (omega-3) fats may also strengthen blood vessel walls, as these are the fats that make up the lipids in the brain and myelin sheathing.

Since 1948, clinicians have been employing diets low in saturated fats when treating multiple sclerosis patients, while researchers strive to find the biochemical links between fat and the disease's pathway.

Researchers attempting to unearth the causes of multiple sclerosis have pinpointed a number of dietary factors based simply on the disease's prevalence around the world.

For example, more cases of multiple sclerosis show up in populations living in higher latitudes, and the highest risk areas include the northern United States and Canada, Great Britain, Scandinavia, northern Europe, New Zealand, and Tasmania. In other words, multiple sclerosis is far more common among people who rely on diets high in saturated fat.

Comparing inland farming communities in Norway to seacoast villages in that country, for instance, has led investigators to conclude that the inland farmers suffered a higher incidence of multiple sclerosis at least partly because they ate greater quantities of saturated animal fat than their seacoast neighbors.

Dr. Roy Swank, professor of neurology at the University of Oregon Medical School, has provided the most successful dietary programs designed to treat multiple sclerosis. As early as 1950, he proposed an association between high levels of dietary fat and the incidence of multiple sclerosis.

In Swank's studies, which were conducted over a period of more than fifteen years, he has found that patients who ate low-fat diets (less than 20 grams a day) are less likely to be disabled by multiple sclerosis attacks. In particular, minimally disabled patients who followed his dietary recommendations deteriorated little if at all.

Some investigators are currently studying whether a deficient intake in certain polyunsaturated fatty acids—so crucial for cell metabolism and healthy cell membranes—might also be an essential link between fats and multiple sclerosis. For example, in a trial using polyunsaturated fatty acids in treating multiple sclerosis, researchers at the Royal Victoria Infirmary of Newcastle, England, have confirmed earlier studies demonstrating that manipulating and supplementing dietary intake of "good" fats—the omega-3 and omega-6 polyunsaturated fatty acids—can alter the percentages of fatty acids in the blood serum of multiple sclerosis patients.

In light of the research conducted so far on using nutrition to manage multiple sclerosis, we recommend the following:

- Decrease your saturated fat intake to no more than 5–10 grams per day by opting for vegetarian protein from beans, grains, and vegetables.
- Increase your omega-3 and GLA omega-6 fats to 50 grams a day by eating more fish and fish oils, particularly those containing EPA and DHA, flaxseed oil, and borage oil.
- Following the basic nutritional principles outlined earlier in this book.

## Nutritional Supplements You Should Begin Taking Now

### • Build Up That Myelin with the Essential Fats: DHA and Oils

Remember that the important omega-3 fatty acid, DHA, is involved in a number of cellular functions and essential to good communication between nerve cells. In addition, omega-3 fatty acids are important ingredients for your body's production of prostaglandins, some of which serve to tone down immune response.

Certainly, additional research needs to be completed before we can be completely certain of the role fatty acids play in protecting against multiple sclerosis. However, there is ample evidence on the table now to suggest that omega-3 fatty acids such as DHA should get top billing for their contributions to building up central nervous system lipids and discouraging the formation of certain prostaglandins capable of triggering inflammatory processes and overall cellular malfunction.

Some fatty acids have the potential to build up damaged myelin and help bring the immune system back under control. In addition, studies designed to examine the role that fatty acids play in modulating immune system response demonstrate that omega-3 fatty acids have a significant modulating effect on the immune system.

We therefore recommend that multiple sclerosis patients supplement their intake of fatty acids with DHA, flaxseed oil, and primrose or borage oils.

**RECOMMENDED DAILY DOSES:**

| | |
|---|---|
| DHA | 300 mg, with a meal. Look for the trademarked Neuromins™ from Martek Biosciences Corporation. |
| Flaxseed oil | 1 tbsp with a meal (cold-pressed, organic preferred, stored in refrigerator) |
| Primrose or borage oil | 2 g with a meal (cold-pressed, organic preferred) |

## PS: A Way to Reduce Tumor Necrosis Factor

As we mentioned earlier, TNF (tumor necrosis factor) is a potent cytokine, one of the most tireless advance soldiers of the immune system. As a pro-inflammatory substance, it plays a crucial role in the development and debilitating progress of multiple sclerosis by creating passageways for crusading macrophages to barge across the blood-brain barrier and attack myelin. Multiple sclerosis patients have elevated levels of TNF in various organs of their bodies during acute attacks, and higher levels of TNF overall than people who do not have the disease.

Today, researchers are using this information to investigate the potential benefits of a variety of substances heralded for their anti-TNF activity. These include the phospholipid phosphatidylserine.

One of the essential lipids in cell membranes, phosphatidylserine is a safe, over-the-counter substance that definitely reduces levels of the TNF cytokine. Animal studies conducted by Dr. Cedric Raine and his colleagues at Albert Einstein College of Medicine reveal that this phospholipid protects against "experimental autoimmune encephalomyelitis," or EAE, an animal model for multiple sclerosis. EAE models multiple sclerosis because it, too, is an acute inflammatory disease of the central nervous system induced by sensitization to the molecular components of myelin.

In EAE, as in multiple sclerosis, the cytokine mediator TNF charges to battle, causing inflammation and paving the way for macrophages to reach the brain. Recent experiments show that administering extra doses of phosphatidylserine, the phospholipid normally present in cell membranes, can actually reduce the levels of TNF in mice.

In addition, phosphatidylserine may also inhibit the overzealous production of fighter T cells that can contribute to the progression of diseases like EAE and multiple sclerosis. We recommend that all multiple sclerosis patients incorporate a PS supplement into their diets.

*RECOMMENDED DOSE:* 300 mg daily of phosphatidylserine. Look for the trademarked Leci-PS™ from Lucas Meyer.

## Antioxidants: Protecting Cells Subjected to Oxidative Stress

Recall that one of the major mechanisms of injury in cells is oxidative stress, and that oxidative stress is increased when the immune system mobilizes and causes our cells to metabolize more oxygen and spin off greater numbers of oxygen free radicals desperately searching for electrons. While these free radicals accomplish their goal of destroying invaders, they may also damage healthy cells in the process, tearing apart cell membranes and dissolving valuable genetic material.

Cell membrane destruction may result in cellular death. This oxidative stress death warrant may have a greater impact on brain cells because of their constant high rate of oxygen consumption and high numbers of mitochondria, the cellular energy factories our bodies depend on to convert glucose into energy.

A number of studies with multiple sclerosis patients have demonstrated that they experience higher levels of lipid oxidation during attacks. For instance, French researchers reporting in a 1996 *Journal of Neuroimmunology* article tested multiple sclerosis patients for antibodies directed against ten fatty acids and found that these patients had significantly elevated levels of antibodies to those fatty acids. They concluded that, in multiple sclerosis, the cell membranes are being attacked by the immune system, a factor that may arise because the membranes have already been battered by oxidative processes.

In short, then, patients with multiple sclerosis may suffer from increased lipid oxidation that is potentially damaging to the myelin sheath so essential to conducting messages along nerve cells. Basically, free radicals amplify injury to myelin by disrupting its fatty acid components.

From this, we conclude that incorporating antioxidant supplements into the diet as a way of preventing lipid oxidation is a key step to protecting against multiple sclerosis attacks. Here, we list a select group of antioxidants pertinent to multiple sclerosis patients.

> **RECOMMENDED DOSE:** A complete advanced antioxidant formula, taken in the amounts prescribed on the label.

## • Glutathione Boosters: Strengthen Myelin with Lipoic Acid, NAC, and Selenium

It is essential that all multiple sclerosis patients begin building up their levels of glutathione from the time of diagnosis.

Examining levels of glutathione peroxidase (GSH-Px) in patients with multiple sclerosis reveals reduced levels in those patients. In one Scandinavian study, multiple sclerosis has been associated with low levels of lymphocyte glutathione peroxidase. When the patients were treated with glutathione, investigators discovered that levels of this essential myelin-strengthening ingredient rose by a factor of five after just a few weeks.

Our nutritional protocol suggests increasing the patient's intake of glutathione, which is necessary for the body's production of GSH-Px. Glutathione enzymes protect proteins and vitamins C and E, thereby warding off oxidative damage and the toxic compounds existing in the environment around us.

While adding glutathione directly to the diet is a logical approach, it is not the best one, as glutathione is poorly absorbed. Nor is it possible to give large amounts of L-cysteine, its precursor, since that compound is toxic in high doses.

Therefore, the best approach to increasing glutathione production in the body is to supplement the diet with lipoic acid (ALA), n-acetyl-cysteine (NAC), and selenium.

ALA has proven to be an important antioxidant compound, in that it regenerates vitamins C and E in cells and is a powerful free radical scavenger. Additionally, ALA has the potential to remove potentially toxic metals from the bloodstream—an important therapeutic aspect in multiple sclerosis and in many other neurological diseases.

The ability of NAC to increase cellular glutathione and reduce tumor necrosis factor levels has been well studied in animal models. In one Israeli study, researchers examined the ability of oral doses of the oxidant-scavenger NAC to halt the progress of EAE, the animal virus model so similar to multiple sclerosis, and discovered that NAC substantially slowed down the development of the virus in mice.

NAC supplements enhance the levels of glutathione in the cells, plasma, and lungs, and influences the immune system by lowering levels of cytokines—all important for multiple sclerosis patients.

**RECOMMENDED DAILY DOSES:**

| | |
|---|---|
| NAC (n-acetyl-cysteine) | 1 g, on an empty stomach |
| Vitamin C | Up to 5 g taken in divided doses throughout the day, with meals |
| Lipoic Acid | 200 mg, with meals |
| Selenium | 200 mcg, with meals (Do not exceed this dose.) |

## Vitamin B12: Protecting Myelin from Breakdown

Both multiple sclerosis and vitamin B12 deficiency may result in the demyelination of nerve sheaths. Symptoms common to both a deficiency in B12 and multiple sclerosis include visual loss, abnormal sensory responses, and abnormal reflexes. There are two key differences between a B12 deficiency and multiple sclerosis, however. First of all, a severe B12 deficiency may lead to a disruption of myelin synthesis, while multiple sclerosis results in the breakdown of myelin. Second, a vitamin B12 deficiency is easily remedied with vitamin supplements, which is why this deficiency must be ruled out in making a diagnosis of multiple sclerosis.

Often, however, individuals with multiple sclerosis also have a vitamin B12 deficiency. Although the extent and mechanism of the association between the two has yet to be determined, British investigator Dr. E. H. Reynolds notes in the *Archives of Neurology* that vitamin B12 injections have been used for over thirty years in treating multiple sclerosis, with mild to marked neurologic benefit to those patients.

There may be a problem with vitamin B12 binding or transport associated with multiple sclerosis. At the very least, vitamin B12 is important for building and strengthening myelin, and any B12 deficiency may aggravate multiple sclerosis or impede recovery.

Although more studies need to be done to determine the exact role that B12 plays in building up myelin sheath on damaged nerve fibers, we recommend that patients explore a combination of injectable and oral sublingual B12 supplements.

RECOMMENDED DAILY DOSE: 1000 mcg, taken sublingually (under the tongue).

## Threonine: Fighting Spasticity

The amino acid threonine is a precursor of glycine synthesis in the spinal cord and essential to maintaining a healthy central nervous system. As early as 1980, investigators began examining the value of threonine supplements in treating multiple sclerosis. They discovered that administering threonine helped some patients to reduce spasticity and improve mobility, particularly of their lower limbs.

Also, in a study conducted by Dr. Stephen Hauser at Massachusetts General Hospital, multiple sclerosis patients treated with threonine showed improvement. Best of all, these patients did not suffer the side effects experienced by those who took antispasticity drugs, which may cause increased motor weakness and sedation.

RECOMMENDED DOSE: 2 g of threonine daily, divided into two doses and taken on an empty stomach.

## Magnesium: An Important Accessory Nutrient

Japanese investigators have reported that the average magnesium content in the central nervous system (CNS) tissue and visceral organs of patients with multiple sclerosis is significantly lower than in patients without the disease, especially in the CNS white matter.

A chronic magnesium deficiency reduces the number of lymphocytes, especially the T cells, which can result in impairing the immune system. Magnesium is also essential in the development, structure, and stability of myelin.

RECOMMENDED DOSE: Up to 600 mg daily, in divided doses. Look for a fully reacted mineral chelate for maximum absorption and utilization.

## What Other Neuroimmunomodulating Medical Therapies Should You Discuss with Your Health Care Practitioner?

• Reflag the Myelin and Fool the Immune System

Our new understanding of the biochemical processes involved in multiple sclerosis has led to a number of promising treatment studies. One strategy has been to look for ways to reflag the myelin so that it doesn't fall under the threat of friendly fire by the immune system. The two substances that satisfy this approach are myelin basic protein and copolymer-1. An additional substance, MP4, is in early clinical trials for its potential in this regard as well.

In one study conducted by Harvard Medical School investigators, multiple sclerosis patients treated with myelin basic protein suffered no side effects to the drug and many of them suffered fewer multiple sclerosis attacks. Currently, a multicenter, double-blind, placebo-controlled study with over 500 patients is being conducted to assess the benefits of treating multiple sclerosis with oral doses of myelin basic protein.

In other studies, physicians have discovered that copolymer-1 is also effective in reversing the process of molecular mimicry that results in myelin breakdown. The copolymer-1 compound was developed at the Weissman Institute in Israel. It is composed of four amino acids with the same sequence and length as myelin basic protein.

When physicians treated over 250 multiple sclerosis patients with copolymer-1 in a trial involving researchers and patients from eleven different universities, they found that this drug reduced the relapse rate. In fact, over half of the patients taking copolymer-1 were relapse-free, and few patients suffered side effects.

The principle in using copolymer-1 to treat multiple sclerosis is simple: When the immune system identifies copolymer-1 as a myelin basic protein, its warriors are distracted from attacking the myelin itself. The drug resembles myelin basic protein so much, in fact, that it may actually inhibit the activation of certain types of warrior T cells in the immune system.

## • Reduce Immune System Response by Lowering Gamma Interferon Production

Another potential strategy for alleviating multiple sclerosis attacks involves using beta interferons. Interferons are naturally occurring proteins produced by the immune system. Beta interferon has been advocated for use in treating multiple sclerosis because of its antiviral activity and its ability to boost the immune system. In fact, it is produced within the human body naturally in cases of inflammation.

Avonex, a genetically produced beta interferon identical to human interferon, has been approved by the FDA to treat relapsing multiple sclerosis. Recently, a multicenter study showed that Avonex decreases the frequency and extent of attacks in patients with multiple sclerosis.

The drawback to treating multiple sclerosis with interferons lies in the significant side effects that some patients experience, including severe flu symptoms and depression.

## Putting It All Together

One of the first steps we took in treating Regina was to start her on a low-fat diet and encourage her to begin incorporating vegetarian protein from beans, grains, and vegetables. We also boosted Regina's intake of essential fatty acids with supplements of 300 mg PS and 400 mg DHA, as well as upping her antioxidant activity with a complete antioxidant supplement. To build up her natural cellular production of glutathione, we also added supplements of 200 mg lipoic acid, 500 mg NAC, and 200 mcg selenium daily.

Probably just as important to Regina's health was her ability to manage stress in her life—an essential step in preventing further multiple sclerosis attacks and in getting herself back on her feet following her divorce. Regina joined a support group for single parents at her church, and she is now practicing bio-feedback and meditation after a series of stress reduction classes at the hospital. After more than two years, Regina has not experienced another multiple sclerosis attack.

Now that you have an overview of multiple sclerosis and how it affects the very structure, function, and biochemical metabolism of the brain–immune system connection, you are probably eager to get started—or to help someone you love begin—investigating a complete treatment protocol.

Here is our summary guideline for treatment.

*Daily Nutritional Supplements*

PS (Look for Leci-PS™        300 mg, with food
    material from Lucas
    Meyer)

| | |
|---|---|
| DHA (Look for Neuromins™ DHA material from Martek Biosciences Corporation) | 300 mg, with food |
| Flaxseed oil (organic, cold-pressed, store in refrigerator) | 2 tbsp, with food |
| Antioxidants | A complete antioxidant supplement, taken according to the amounts prescribed on the label |
| Lipoic acid | 200 mg, with food |
| NAC (n-acetyl-cysteine) | 1 g, on an empty stomach |
| B12 | 1000 mg of a sublingual (under the tongue) supplement |
| Threonine | 2 g, on an empty stomach |
| Selenium | 200 mcg, with food (This amount should not be exceeded. Therefore, you will need to add up the amounts of selenium you get from your multiple vitamins and antioxidant formula.) |

*Medications Summary*

Beta interferons

Copolymer I

Myelin basic protein (Currently available in health food stores, a patent is now pending on myelin basic protein and it may soon be available only by prescription.)

# CHAPTER 8

# AMYOTROPHIC LATERAL SCLEROSIS
## (LOU GEHRIG'S DISEASE)

Leonard, an avid golfer, usually left his dental practice early on Wednesdays to get in a round with his partner at the public course just outside of town. It was there, one fine May afternoon, that he noticed he couldn't flex his ankle properly. Leonard attributed this symptom to an old sprain which sometimes acted up in damp weather.

However, Leonard's ankle was no less stiff by Christmas, and he was beginning to notice that his hands, too, were so lame that he had trouble buttoning his shirts. What's more, he felt tired all the time.

"You're too young to act so old," Leonard's wife teased, until he finally relented and saw their family physician.

Leonard's doctor was more concerned than Leonard had expected him to be. He immediately referred Leonard to a neurologist, who performed a complete physical exam and discovered that Leonard showed brisk, abnormal reflexes in his lower extremities.

The neurologist asked Leonard to come in to the hospital for several laboratory and radiographic tests, including a spinal fluid test, a blood test, a magnetic resonance imaging (MRI) test on his brain and spinal cord, and an EMG (electromyogram) to measure the electrical activity in Leonard's nerves and muscles.

These tests confirmed the neurologist's suspicions. He diagnosed amyotrophic lateral sclerosis (ALS), and set up an appointment with Leonard and his wife to discuss treatment options.

## Amyotrophic Lateral Sclerosis: An Overview

A progressive neuromuscular disease, amyotrophic lateral sclerosis (ALS) is sometimes referrred to as "Lou Gehrig's disease" for the famous baseball star afflicted with this condition. Other celebrities to be diagnosed with ALS include the musician Charles Mingus and astrophysicist Stephen Hawking.

Nearly 1 out of every 50,000 people worldwide is diagnosed with ALS each year, with over 5,000 new cases reported in the United States annually. Of the U.S. population living today, about 300,000 will die from ALS, with 35,000 Americans suffering from the disease at any one time.

Nearly twice as many men are affected by ALS as women. While most people are diagnosed with the disease in their mid-fifties, ALS has been reported in teenagers and in much older patients.

The incidence of ALS is about equal to that of multiple sclerosis. However, people diagnosed with multiple sclerosis may live for decades with the disease, while those with ALS typically die of the disease between two and five years after diagnosis. ALS places a great financial burden on families, as all people with ALS eventually become bedridden. Care can amount to more than $200,000 annually.

Thankfully, the outlook for people with ALS is now brighter than ever before. Research conducted over the past decades has finally begun to shed light on the actual mechanisms involved in ALS, which was first described in 1869 by the noted French neurologist Jean-Martin Charcot. In fact, in 1996 the first drug ever to prove effective in treating ALS was approved by the FDA.

More promising ALS treatments are in the offing as we continue to develop our understanding of the disease's pathways and mechanisms. Now, up to 10 percent of those with ALS can be expected to survive more than ten years after diagnosis.

While researchers have not yet fully defined the causes or

pathways of ALS, we now know that the disease attacks specific motor neurons in the brain and spinal cord. These nerve cells are among the body's largest and extend from the brain to the spinal cord, and from the spinal cord to muscles throughout the body.

In patients with ALS, the motor neurons die and the brain's ability to control muscle movement dies with them. Hence the name "amyotrophic," which comes from the Greek for "no muscle nourishment." The word "lateral" refers to the fact that most of these nerve cells die in the spinal cord of ALS patients, leading to "sclerosis," or scarring.

As a result of losing so many motor neurons, ALS patients eventually become totally paralyzed, though their minds remain unaffected by the disease. Both experimental animal and clinical studies suggest that the key causes of ALS are an overabundance of glutamate, the neurotransmitter that nerve cells rely on to transmit signals, and excessive oxidative damage to cells.

In essence, then, it seems that ALS, like Alzheimer's, Parkinson's, and many other neurological illnesses, may in large part be caused by a series of biochemical events leading to excessive free radical damage to healthy brain cells.

In this chapter, we discuss ALS from the onset of symptoms to diagnosis, beginning with what we know about the disease's effects on motor neurons at the most basic, molecular level.

At our chapter's conclusion, we offer a complete treatment plan for ALS based on the most current information available on diet, nutritional supplements, and medications.

## What Goes Wrong in ALS, and Why?

Essentially, ALS is characterized by dying motor nerve cells in the brain—called the "upper motor neurons"—and in the spine, where the "lower motor neurons" are located. As the disease progresses, the long nerve cells that go from the top of the skull to the spinal cord and from the spinal cord to the limbs progressively deteriorate, eventually leaving the patient completely paralyzed.

At present, scientists can predict no specific similarities of all people diagnosed with ALS, so the cause remains unknown. Physicians currently classify ALS according to how nerve damage progresses and whether or not it is inherited. The categories of ALS include:

1. Classical ALS, which affects over two-thirds of all people with ALS and is characterized by the deterioration of both upper and lower motor nerve cells.
2. Primary lateral sclerosis, which causes only the upper motor neurons to deteriorate.
3. Progressive muscular atrophy, in which only the lower motor neurons degenerate.
4. Progressive bulbar palsy, a condition that begins with difficulties in chewing, swallowing, and speech.
5. Familial ALS, so named because it affects more than one member in the same family.

## • *Families with ALS Provide a Genetic Clue*

There are two ways of developing ALS. One way is inherited. The other is random. In the genetic form, each child of a parent with ALS has a 50 percent chance of inheriting the ALS gene. Everyone who inherits the gene is eventually diagnosed with the disease. Although only 5–10 percent of patients with ALS inherited the disease, familial ALS has led scientists to uncover genetic clues that may prove useful in detailing the disease's pathways in all types of ALS.

In 1991, for example, a team of researchers linked ALS to chromosome 21. Just two years later, this same group of investigators identified a defective SOD1 (superoxide dismutase enzyme) gene on that chromosome as the culprit responsible for many cases of familial ALS.

Why is the SOD enzyme so important to your body that a defective version of it could lead to this devastating illness?

In healthy brains, this enzyme performs a crucial maintenance task by mopping up peroxynitrite, the highly toxic free radical produced as a result of excessive levels of the glutamate neurotransmitter (see below).

Peroxynitrite is normally released in abundance by white

blood cells during the course of immune system battles—as in viral or bacterial infections—and plays a powerful role in immune system inflammation. If the SOD enzyme is ineffective in clearing the brain of that toxic free radical, however, the destructive effect to healthy cells is equivalent to turning a herd of bulls loose in a china shop, with free radicals causing rampant destruction.

In one recent study, for example, the brains of patients with ALS were analyzed for glutathione peroxidase and superoxide dismutase, two of the enzymes so critical for inhibiting free radical destruction. This study demonstrated that the brains of patients who died of ALS had significantly reduced amounts of these enzymes, suggesting that they had less protection against free radical attacks on healthy brain cells. Meanwhile, researchers at the University of California have concluded that oxidative reactions in the brains of patients with a defective SOD gene initiates the domino effect of neuropathologic changes among those with ALS.

Although SOD1 mutations have been discovered in only a minority of all patients—about 30 percent of the patients among those with familial ALS—this landmark discovery is certain to lead to a clearer understanding of the disease. That's because ALS progresses in essentially the same manner even in the 98 percent of the patients without the mutation.

### • Too Much Glutamate Causes Too Much Excitement

Some natural substances stimulate brain cells. Glutamate, the amino acid neurotransmitter responsible for exciting neurons to fire off messages, is one of them. Glutamate's normal interactions with specific membrane receptors in brain cells are responsible for driving many important neurological functions. These include cognition, memory, movement, and sensation, as Harvard researchers have reported in *Mechanisms of Disease*.

However, as in the case of so many neurotransmitters, just a little too much of a good thing can throw the brain's complex communication network completely off kilter. When too much glutamate lingers outside cells and binds with neuron receptors, neurotransmitters are triggered to fire more than they should.

Essentially, the brain cells then wear themselves out and die from exhaustion as a result.

Glutamate has been implicated in a variety of brain diseases. This is because excessive activation of glutamate receptors—called "excitotoxicity"—serves as a final common pathway leading to neuron death.

Researchers at Baylor College of Medicine and other institutions are attempting to identify exactly what happens to cause extracellular glutamate to build up toxic levels, and what governs selective motor neuron death in ALS. (Several other studies have demonstrated that patients have elevated glutamate in their cerebral spinal fluid.) This indicates that they are unable to metabolize glutamate normally.

## • What Could Cause Patients with ALS to Have Too Much Glutamate in the First Place?

As we have discussed, patients with ALS suffer from high levels of glutamate. In fact, research has uncovered evidence revealing that glutamate levels are higher in the blood serum and cerebrospinal fluid of people with ALS than in those without the disease.

The leading theory about why patients with ALS suffer from toxic levels of glutamate throws the spotlight on astrocytes, the brain's star-shaped cells that normally sop up extra neurotransmitter molecules around neurons to protect them from overstimulation.

Much as unwanted garbage collects if a city's trash collectors go on strike, patients with ALS may suffer when astrocytes fail to adequately pick up glutamate and transport it away from neurons. The question, then, is why should the astrocytes go on strike and fail to perform their clean-up duties in the brain?

As with anyone who goes on strike, astrocytes may be reacting to poor working conditions or low "pay." Glutamate uptake by astrocytes requires an enormous amount of energy expenditure, as well as a key enzyme known as GLT-1. A careful analysis of the glutamate transport system in patients with ALS has demonstrated a selective loss of GLT-1.

According to a number of studies performed by leading ALS research Dr. Jeffrey Rothstein and his colleagues at Johns Hopkins University, this is probably due to damage by free radicals or environmental toxins. Currently, scientists at the University of British Columbia, UCLA, and the University of California, Irvine, are among those investigating further the reasons for astrocytes falling down on the job of glutamate cleanup.

Besides a deficiency in GLT-1, astrocytes may be subjected to poor working conditions as a result of being exposed to methylmercury and other toxic metals. Methylmercury is a common contaminant in industrial society that can be highly hazardous to brain cells—principally because it inhibits the uptake of glutamate by astrocyte cleanup cells. It may be one of the poisons causing the destruction of the GLT-1 protein.

Does heavy metal accumulation in neurons automatically mark those cells for eventual degeneration?

The answer seems to be that it does, and that motor neurons, in particular, possess a selective affinity for certain toxic metals.

The concept that toxic metals may be linked to ALS has been extensively studied, with continuing reports of ALS-like syndromes associated with toxic metal intake and exposure. Some toxic metals, such as mercury, lead, and aluminum, are such ubiquitous environmental pollutants that the stage is set for long-term, low-level exposure for many of us, as the half-lives for most toxic metals in the body are very long.

For example, chronic dietary deficiencies of calcium and magnesium, when combined with excess intake of aluminum and manganese, have been implicated in the high incidence of ALS among people living in the Western Pacific. This is most likely because poor metabolism of calcium and magnesium is implicated in the inability to displace aluminum out of body tissue among ALS patients.

Japanese studies have revealed that ALS patients suffered from low serum selenium and mercury levels. While a low serum mercury level may seem to be desirable, it reflects greater stores in body tissue, where it exerts its toxic effect. Additionally, it is well known that selenium can decrease mercury toxicity because of selenium's role in promoting glutathione enzyme detoxification. Therefore, mercury exposure and adequate selenium intake should both be assessed in patients with ALS.

Other Western Pacific studies have demonstrated that chronic dietary deficiencies of calcium and magnesium, with excess intakes of aluminum and manganese, are also associated with a high incidence of ALS. Additional studies detecting elevated aluminum levels in the CNS tissue of people with ALS also reveal increased calcified material, similar to calcium.

To date, investigators are honing in on various antioxidants with the potential to act as free radical scavengers able to confer protection against heavy metal toxicity. These include lipoic acid, glutathione, selenium, and n-acetyl-cysteine, which we will discuss in the nutritional section at the end of this chapter.

### • What Actually Causes Cells to Die, If They Are Overstimulated by Too Much Glutamate?

In recent years, researchers around the world have been investigating this puzzling paradox: Why have our brains evolved with such extraordinary vulnerability to our own neurotransmitters? And what events actually lead to the abnormal accumulation of such neurotransmitters?

In the case of glutamate, neurons swell and die just a few hours after exposure. Glutamate-related neuron death goes something like this: The excess of glutamate causes neurons to fire too often. This excessive neuron stimulation provokes a rise in intracellular sodium, which in turn interferes with the cell's necessary energy stores of glucose and oxygen.

In addition, the brain cells caused to fire too often by the presence of an overabundance of glutamate also end up allowing too much calcium to cross into the cell through membrane channels. While intracellular calcium is essential for a number of processes, too much calcium inside a cell can trigger harmful reactions, including the activation of various cell-busting enzymes. One of these enzymes can even lead to the production of arachidonic acid, the deadly substance discussed earlier in this book.

In the case of ALS, arachidonic acid perpetuates cell damage by further inhibiting the uptake of glutamate by the brain's astrocytes. Free radicals formed as a result of arachidonic acid metabolism can inflict further damage on cells.

What's more, when receptors are stimulated because too much glutamate is hammering on brain cell membranes, nitric oxide and superoxide may be produced. Together, these substances may react to form one of the free radicals that serves a death warrant to cells: peroxynitrite.

In essence, then, excessive glutamate in the brain actually causes motor neurons to self-destruct through a combination of sodium and calcium imbalances, protein breakdown, and free radical damage.

Now, researchers are looking into ways to stop this biochemical domino effect before it starts.

Because the glutamate neurotransmitter must "match up" with certain receptors on receiving neurons to succeed in stimulating those neurons, investigators are now exploring ways to block those receptors. If those receptors can be prevented from receiving glutamate stimulation, then we may one day successfully protect cells against death by exhaustion.

Another protective strategy is to block the release of excitatory glutamate from brain cells in the first place. Riluzole, the first drug approved for patients with ALS, has proven effective in doing just that. We will discuss this drug later, in our section on ALS medications.

### • Why Are More Men Diagnosed with ALS than Women?

Investigators are currently investigating possible reasons to explain why more men are diagnosed with ALS than women. One theory concerns DHEA.

DHEA (dehydroepiandrosterone), a natural hormone produced by the brain, has been closely scrutinized by scientists in recent years for its potential for everything from restoring memory to delaying aging, and has been shown to reduce body fat and to protect against cardiovascular mortality among men.

In fact, DHEA is naturally abundant in the brain, and is important for its "neurotrophic" factor. That is, DHEA is one of the nourishing agents that neurons depend on for growth and survival. Other important neuron growth factors, as we will see in our section on nutrition, include brain-derived nerve growth factor and insulin-like growth factor. All of these serve as "fertilizer" for brain cells, allowing them to grow strong and communicate efficiently.

The higher incidence of ALS in men may reflect the fact that DHEA levels in men start out much higher than in women. DHEA levels peak in adolescence, however, and decline with age among most men, so that production of that hormone at age sixty-five is just 10–20 percent of what it was at age twenty.

Researchers reporting in a 1995 issue of *Muscle and Nerve* postulate that the rapid decline of this hormone among men may be an important factor in causing more men to be diagnosed with ALS than women. It may be that men need more DHEA than women do, and the age related decline affects them more adversely.

# A Complete Blueprint for Care

If you or a loved one is diagnosed with ALS, the most important step you can take is to work with your physician to discuss both standard and research treatment protocols. Because of the disease's rapid progress, it is essential to take action immediately toward preventing neuron degeneration and maintaining the highest quality of life possible.

Patients with ALS suffer from inefficient glutamate metabolism resulting in a state of neuron excitotoxicity and excessive free radical damage to motor neurons.

Here, we present an aggressive protocol of nutritional neuroimmunomodulators with the potential to address these conditions. Our treatment strategies include adding growth factors, antioxidants, and other substances tailored to nourish motor neuron growth, inhibit glutamate release from cells, block neuron receptors from binding with glutamate, and stop free radicals in their tracks.

As the disease progresses, we offer patients a combination of counseling, medications, speech therapy, and assistive devices as necessary.

TABLE **6**
_____

## ALS: THE STEPS LEADING TO MOTOR NEURON DEATH

1. In the case of familial ALS, a defective form of the SOD1 gene impairs the brain's natural ability to cleanse itself of toxic superoxide free radicals, causing nerve cells to rapidly degenerate.

2. For some patients with ALS, exposure to toxins such as methylmercury may lead to the brain's inability to properly metabolize glutamate, the brain's key excitatory neurotransmitter.

3. For all patients with ALS, the brain's ability to metabolize glutamate is faulty, possibly as a result of astrocyte cells being unable to successfully clean up the brain.

4. Because it is an excitatory neurotransmitter with the ability to trigger cells to fire, an excessive amount of glutamate in the brain can cause cells to fire too often and die.

5. Motor neurons die off progressively, causing eventual paralysis and death.

## When Should You Suspect ALS?

ALS is a difficult disease to diagnose, as it affects everyone differently. However, some of the most common early symptoms of the disease include muscle twitches and cramping, especially in the hands and feet.

Patients in the early stages of ALS may also notice generalized muscle weakness and fatigue, and may discover that it is difficult to project their voices. Their speech, too, may be affected, and sound "thick" or slurred.

As the disease becomes more severe—over the course of anywhere from just a few months to several years, depending on the individual—patients may have difficulty chewing and swallowing, as the nerves degenerate, resulting in weight loss. They will also have trouble breathing.

Severe pain is not a typical symptom of ALS, nor is there any impairment in thinking or memory.

## Diagnosing ALS: No Single Test

In diagnosing ALS, your neurologist will perform a complete physical exam and take a medical history. Two of the diseases most commonly misdiagnosed as ALS include:

- *Cervical spondylosis,* a degeneration of the spinal cord due to chronic arthritis. Typically, the diagnosis can be confirmed through an MRI.
- *Multifocal motor neuropathy,* a disease that specifically strikes lower motor neurons without upper motor neuron symptoms. In this case, the diagnosis can be clarified with an EMG (see below) and with a test for antibodies to motor neurons.

It is essential to rule out these two ALS-mimicking diseases, as they each require unique treatments.

In completing a lab workup to diagnose ALS definitively, your neurologist should request blood tests, a spinal fluid test, an EMG (electromyogram) to measure the electrical activity in your nerves and muscles, and an MRI (magnetic resonance imaging) to produce a complete image of the body without using x-rays.

### • Check for Heavy Metal Toxicity

Based on studies we cited earlier in this chapter on the possible detrimental effects to motor neurons of heavy metals such as mercury, iron, and aluminum, we recommend that all patients diagnosed with ALS consider being tested for heavy metal toxicity.

Some physicians will recommend blood testing to do this. However, if blood tests are normal and metal toxicity is still suspected, your health care practitioner may recommend a urine test performed before and after chelation. (Chelation involves administering an oral agent to increase urinary excretion of a metal.)

If such toxicity exists, certain nutritional agents can be incorporated into the daily regimen to alleviate the metal burden in the body (see below).

## The First Step to Take: Ensure a Nutritious Diet

In research conducted at the University of Chicago Hospital's ALS Outpatient Clinic, clinicians discovered the following:

- About 70 percent of the patients suffered from calorie intake that fell below RDA guidelines, leading to a loss in body weight among a quarter of the patients.
- At least 25 percent of the patients suffered from moderate to severe malnutrition.
- Fifteen percent of the patients had elevated serum glucose.
- About 20 percent showed elevated cholesterol levels.

Since not all patients with ALS lose weight, we can conclude that weight loss is not just due to a loss in muscle mass. Rather, patients with ALS should be examined with an eye toward proper caloric intake, a physical ability to prepare food and feed oneself, and psychological well-being, as all of these factors contribute to the state of nourishment.

While no specific diet exists for those diagnosed with ALS, patients can help maintain quality of life by following our recommendations in the two-step Brain Wellness Plan presented earlier in this book. Good nutrition can provide patients with more energy and a better sense of well-being, as well as strengthen the immune system.

Therefore, one of the first steps we recommend is determining early on whether any nutritional problems are present so that your nutritionist or health care provider can institute appropriate nutritional interventions. Patients with ALS may need special help with swallowing problems, either through formulas or blenderized foods, for example.

## • Ease Constipation with Fluids and Dietary Fiber

ALS patients typically have problems with constipation owing to weakened gastrointestinal muscle control. In addition to incorporating insoluble types of fiber into the diet by eating rice bran and whole grain breads, crackers, and cereals, we suggest that patients with ALS drink a minimum of eight glasses of water daily. Patients should also consider adding supplements of Miller's bran and psyllium fiber as directed by a nutritionist. Additionally, individuals with ALS should add sufficient fruits and vegetables to their diets as outlined in *The Brain Wellness Plan* dietary guidelines.

## • Avoid Glutamine

As we have seen, the amino acid glutamate is a potentially potent central nervous system toxin in ALS. Now, animal studies conducted by researchers at the Arkansas National Center for Toxicological Research have demonstrated that glutamine, which can serve as an important source of nitrogen and energy for most healthy individuals, has the undesirable effect of enhancing the release of glutamate from brain cells.

This study has important implications for patients with ALS, naturally, since motor neurons are already compromised by excessive levels of glutamate. We therefore strongly discourage patients from taking any glutamine supplements.

## • Avoid Iron

University of Kentucky researchers investigating the roles of aluminum, calcium, and iron have discovered that individuals with ALS had consistently elevated iron levels in their spinal neurons. These investigators concluded that the elevation of iron in the CNS was significant in the pathogenesis of motor neuron degeneration primarily because high iron levels may enhance the spinoff of deadly free radicals within specific cells.

Based on these and other studies examining iron levels in

ALS patients, we recommend that individuals with ALS avoid any nutritional supplements that contain iron.

### • What about Branched Chain Amino Acids?

The branched chain amino acids (BCAA) leucine, isoleucine, and valine are essential amino acids primarily involved in stress, energy, and muscle metabolism. With respect to muscle, the BCAAs are directly used as energy sources to stimulate protein synthesis.

In the past decade, researchers have been examining the association between BCAAs and the muscle wasting that is a hallmark of ALS. For example, in a study published in *Lancet,* one researcher showed that supplementing the diets of ALS patients with BCAAs resulted in a significant improvement in muscle strength.

Unfortunately, other studies have not duplicated these successful results. In fact, one study had to be discontinued when researchers noted that subjects taking BCAA experienced an excess mortality. What's more, another investigation—this one conducted in a Denmark hospital by researchers Gredal and Moller—revealed that BCAA supplements actually elevated plasma glutamate within forty-five minutes of taking them.

For these reasons, we do not recommend supplementing the diets of ALS individuals with BCAAs, owing to potentially negative effects.

## Nutritional Supplements You Should Begin Taking Now

### • Raise SOD Levels to Beat Back Free Radical Damage

As you learned earlier in this chapter, patients with the familial type of ALS have a genetically impaired SOD (superoxide dismutase) enzyme system. SOD is an enzyme found in most cells in the body, and it is critical as a free radical neutralizer—especially when it comes to stripping the toxic oxygen radical, superoxide, of its power.

The two major types of SOD are Cu/Zn SOD and Mn SOD. Cu/Zn SOD contains the minerals copper and zinc, and protects the cell's cytoplasm. Meanwhile, Mn SOD is activated by manganese and protects the cells' energy factories, the mitochondria.

How can you boost your levels of SOD? In animal studies at Oklahoma State University, researchers measured SOD activity in animals after giving them either inorganic forms of copper, zinc, and magnesium as compared to chelated forms of the minerals. The term "chelated" mineral refers to a process by which a mineral is attached to another substance for the sole purpose of assisting in the absorption and utilization of that mineral. The reason we recommend chelated minerals throughout *The Brain Wellness Plan* is that minerals, in general, are very difficult to absorb, and require assistance in order to be absorbed efficiently.

In the Oklahoma study, investigators discovered that animals taking the chelated minerals showed an increase in SOD of more than 15 percent. Human studies at Purdue University, meanwhile, have demonstrated that SOD activity was boosted by 21 percent in volunteers who received chelated copper alone, while other studies achieved similar results using chelated manganese.

Essentially, then, recent research supports the concept that supplementing the diet of ALS patients with chelated forms of zinc, manganese, and copper will significantly boost the levels of SOD, one of the body's most important free radical fighters. This nutrient may lower the death rate of motor neurons by protecting them from uncontrolled superoxide radicals in particular.

RECOMMENDED DOSES: Look for fully reacted mineral chelates. You may find all three packaged together as a single product.

| | |
|---|---|
| Zinc | 30 mg |
| Copper | 2 mg |
| Manganese | 4 mg |

All these supplements are to be taken daily with food.

## • Add Magnesium to Inhibit Glutamate Release By Cells

In the central nervous system, magnesium serves to inhibit the release of excitatory neurotransmitters such as glutamate. Magnesium may therefore play an important role in protecting brain cells against the calcium-mediated injury that accompanies the too-rapid firing of overstimulated cells. Magnesium does this by blocking the brain cell receptors that could otherwise bind with glutamate.

Furthermore, depressed magnesium levels also result in activating a dangerous enzyme called "phospholipase," which is involved in causing further destruction of brain cells through lipid peroxidation. Studies conducted in the Kii peninsula of Japan—an area where the incidence of ALS is higher than most—revealed that patients suffering from the disease had a significantly low magnesium content in their cerebrospinal fluid. They concluded that low magnesium levels may promote the abnormal metabolism of calcium and magnesium. This may promote an increased vulnerability to the development of ALS.

RECOMMENDED DOSE: Ensure adequate magnesium intake by supplementing the daily diet with 600 mg of chelated magnesium taken in divided amounts with meals.

## • Up Your Antioxidant Intake to Protect Against Toxic Free Radicals

In ALS as in so many other neurological illnesses, oxygen free radicals spun off as a result of cellular breakdown, immune system activation, and the brain's impaired ability to mop up toxic levels of certain neurotransmitters and toxins can lead to cell death.

In addition to adding the full complement of antioxidants through a general supplement, as we suggest in our chapter on The Brain Wellness Plan, there are a number of additional antioxidants which may be of particular benefit to ALS patients.

For example, we emphasize adding the antioxidant coenzyme Q10, since it is capable of pulling apart superoxide so that it can no longer damage delicate cellular machinery. Free radical quenchers, such as ascorbic acid and carotenoids, are also essential backups to the antioxidant arsenal.

Finally, we recommend that patients with ALS add extra amounts of vitamin E, lipoic acid, and polyphenols such as pine bark, grape seed, and green tea extracts as powerful free radical scavengers.

RECOMMENDED DAILY DOSES:
   200 mg coenzyme Q10 with a meal
   4 g ascorbic acid with meals
   25,000 IU carotenoids (look for a combination formula containing all the important carotenoids, such as alpha and beta carotene, lutein, and lycopene)
   400 IU tocopherols with a meal
   60 mg tocotrienols with a meal
   200 mg lipoic acid with a meal
   120 mg of pine bark, grape seed, green tea, or fruit polyphenols

## • NAC: Boost Your Glutathione Production and Decrease Membrane Damage

In other chapters of this book, we have discussed glutathione as one of the body's most important detoxifiers. The glutathione status of any cell is crucial to its health. That's why this natural peptide plays so many roles in battling disease.

For patients with ALS, we recommend boosting glutathione principally because of that amino acid's power as a free radical scavenger, since free radicals rapidly promote the demise of motor neurons. The best way to boost glutathione production is through supplements of NAC (n-acetyl-cysteine) and lipoic acid.

NAC has proven beneficial in decreasing the membrane damage caused by superoxide, even in cells with impaired or absent SOD. In addition, NAC has the ability to reduce the cytokine known as TNF (tumor necrosis factor), which may otherwise promote immune-mediated brain cell injury. And finally, a study reported in *Archives of Neurology* in 1995 revealed that NAC has demonstrated benefits in reducing the rate of disability among ALS patients.

The best food sources for glutathione include acorn squash, asparagus, avocado, grapefruit, orange, potato, strawberries, tomato, watermelon, cauliflower, broccoli, and cantaloupe. In addition, we recommend the glutathione-boosting substances listed below.

*RECOMMENDED DAILY DOSES:*
   200 mg lipoic acid, with a meal
   200 mcg selenium, with a meal
   1 g NAC, taken on an empty stomach

## Auxiliary Nutrients to Consider

• *Creatine: A Potential Muscle Builder*

While no studies exist on using creatine to treat ALS, we suggest that patients consider adding this supplement owing to its important muscle-building powers. Creatine is a nutrient naturally found in our bodies and is made from the amino acids arginine, methionine, and glycine. It has been shown to increase muscle mass through promoting better protein synthesis within muscle fibers. Creatine is also essential for muscle contraction, as it assists in developing ATP, the energy currency for all cells.

*RECOMMENDED DOSAGE:* 5 g daily, on an empty stomach.

• *Threonine: A Key Amino Acid Inhibitor*

You have already seen how glutamate, the excitatory amino acid neurotransmitter, is involved in the breakdown of motor neurons among patients with ALS. One way of inhibiting this overzealous amino acid activity is through supplements of threonine, which has been shown to improve some ALS symptoms.

For example, in a paper published in the *American Family Physician,* clinicians reported that administering threonine daily helped improve speech, energy, and muscle spasticity among those patients. Therefore, we suggest that patients add threonine as part of their overall protocol.

*RECOMMENDED DOSE:* 2 g daily, on an empty stomach.

# Other Neuroimmunomodulating Substances to Discuss with Your Physician

## • *Increase Glutamate Clean-up by Astrocytes*

As we saw earlier, the excessive glutamate accumulated in the brains of patients with ALS may be due to astrocytes "going on strike." To improve the clean-up performance of astrocytes, we should first check heavy metal toxicity. If blood or urine tests show that the body's burden of mercury, lead, or aluminum are too high, the physician may consider treating the patient with chelation therapy. Chelation therapy requires the patient to take an agent that will bind to the metal and cause it to be excreted through the urine. Patients should discuss potential complications of this therapy with a specialist, as it has potentially severe side effects and requires close monitoring. Clinical trials are currently under way to explore the benefits of chelation therapy in ALS patients.

## • *Add Trophic Factors as Fertilizer for Neurons*

As we discussed earlier in this chapter, neuron-nourishing trophic factors such as the hormone DHEA, brain-derived nerve growth factor (BDNF), and insulin-like growth factor in ALS patients may contribute to the improved viability and regenerative capacity of motor neurons.

Growth factors are naturally occurring molecules that promote the survival of motor neurons. A recent study using insulin-like growth factor in patients with ALS revealed that administering that substance significantly delayed disease progress.

DHEA has insulin-like growth factor properties, and is also being explored as a therapy for treating ALS. Most likely, treatment protocols of the future will call for combining BDNF, DHEA, and insulin-like growth factor.

## Medications

### • Riluzole (Rilutek): The Only Approved ALS Drug to Date

As of this writing, the only drug approved for patients with ALS is riluzole, currently marketed under the trade name "Rilutek."

Approved in 1996, the drug is the first prescription treatment for ALS with the demonstrated ability to extend patient survival by blocking the release of glutamate by brain cells. Programs are available to provide long-term support in resolving insurance and reimbursement issues, in an effort to make riluzole available to all patients, regardless of financial status. The drug is generally well tolerated, with the only side effects being nausea, fatigue, and elevated liver enzymes.

Additional drug therapies on the immediate horizon include medications with the ability to interfere with the binding of brain cells to glutamate.

### • Immunophilins: The Potential to Reduce Immune-Mediated Damage

As with so many other neurological illnesses, immune-mediated damage in ALS patients can accelerate neuron death because of the cycle of harmful free radicals produced during inflammation. In the brain, natural substances called immunophilins provide marked protection from the immune system's toxic compounds. FK506, a synthetic immunophilin, is an agent capable of crossing the brain-blood barrier. It is known for its potency in inhibiting the synthesis of nitric oxide, one of the most potentially toxic compounds to brain cells because it serves as a precursor to the deadly peroxynitrite free radical.

Although it is currently approved only as a drug in keeping transplanted organs from being rejected, FK506 is currently under investigation for its potential in treating ALS.

## Putting It All Together

Immediately after diagnosis, Leonard and his wife sought the help of a professional nutritionist to resolve Leonard's weight loss issues through a nutritious, palatable diet. In addition, Leonard began boosting his antioxidant intake through a general supplement combined with the recommended doses of antioxidant boosters described in the chapter. Additionally, we prescribed adequate zinc, copper, and manganese supplements for their ability to induce SOD.

Testing for heavy metal toxicity revealed that Leonard showed no evidence of high mercury levels. We added 600 mg of magnesium to Leonard's daily intake to inhibit glutamate release by cells, and a supplement of DHEA to help nourish Leonard's healthy motor neurons. We also put Leonard on a prescription of riluzole to slow nerve degeneration, and referred Leonard and his family to a regional medical center. He is now participating in a clinical trial using brain-derived nerve growth factor to nourish his brain cells.

Although Leonard's symptoms have progressed over the past three years to the point where he must rely on a walker and occasionally suffers difficulty in swallowing certain foods, he has maintained his upper body strength and remains in good spirits.

Now that you have an overview of ALS and how the disease impacts motor neurons, you are probably anxious to start—or to help someone you love begin—investigating an aggressive treatment protocol.

Here is our summary guideline for treatment.

## Recommended Nutritional Supplements for ALS

Follow the basic healthy eating guidelines in *The Brain Wellness Plan,* and assess individual nutritional needs with a qualified professional. If evidence exists of abnormal glucose tolerance, patients with ALS should incorporate 400 mcg of chelated chromium and 500 mcg of vandyl sulfate.

*Daily Nutritional Supplements*

| | |
|---|---|
| Zinc* | 30 mg, with food |
| Copper* | 2 mg, with food |

| | |
|---|---|
| Manganese* | 4 mg, with food |
| Magnesium* | 600 mg, in divided doses |
| Coenzyme Q10 | 200 mg, with food |
| Ascorbic acid | 4 g, with food |
| Carotenoids | 25,000 IU, with food (Look for a combination formula containing all the important carotenoids, such as alpha and beta carotene, lutein, and lycopene.) |
| Tocopherols | 400 IU, with food |
| Tocotrienols | 60 mg, with food |
| Lipoic acid | 200 mg, with food |
| NAC (n-acetyl-cysteine) | 1500 mg, on an empty stomach |
| Polyphenols | 120 mg (pine bark, grape seed, green tea, or fruit polyphenols) |
| Creatine | 5 g, on an empty stomach |
| Threonine | 2 g, on an empty stomach |

*Look for fully reacted mineral chelates.

*Other Neuroimmunomodulating Substances to Discuss with Your Physician:*

Chelating therapy (in the event of heavy metal toxicity)
Trophic factors such as brain-derived growth factor

*Medications*

FK506
Rilutek (riluzole)

# CHAPTER 9

# ATTENTION DEFICIT HYPERACTIVITY DISORDER

From his first few months of life, Clarissa and Ray knew there was something different about their son Jon. For one thing, he never slept. When other babies his age were sleeping a good ten to twelve hours a night and taking at least one nap every day, Jon was wide awake by 5 A.M. and simply screamed if they tried to get him to rest anytime during the day.

By the time he was two, Jon was a whirling dervish, or as Ray called him, "the human destructo machine," practically climbing the walls. Preschool didn't seem to help. In fact, just getting Jon to sit in the car long enough to buckle his seat belt required all of Clarissa's patience and strength. Once, Jon even managed to wriggle free and jump out of the car before she closed the door, hitting his head on the paved drive. As usual, though, Jon didn't cry. He seemed heedless of danger, no matter how they cautioned him or how many scrapes he bore on his skinny knees and elbows.

In elementary school, Jon's behavior actually worsened. When the teacher tried to read a story, he constantly interrupted. If another child competed with him for a toy, Jon was likely to solve the disagreement with a slap. Clarissa and Ray were worried. If Jon was this out of control now, what would he be like as a teenager?

Jon's preschool teacher recommended that he be evaluated for attention deficit hyperactivity disorder (ADHD). The pediatrician conducted a thorough physical exam, and then referred the family to a child psychiatrist. A battery of behavioral assessment tests confirmed the ADHD diagnosis, and the psychiatrist prescribed Ritalin. However, unconvinced that this was the best solution, Clarissa and Ray sought our opinion.

"There must be other things we can do," they told us. "We really don't want our kid on medication unless there is absolutely no other choice."

## Attention Deficit Hyperactivity Disorder: An Overview

ADHD ranks among the most common neurological disorders among American children, affecting up to 5 percent, or as many as 2 million, U.S. children at any one time.

In fact, in every classroom in the United States you can expect to find at least one child with ADHD. While it is not itself a specific learning disability, ADHD can interfere with concentration and attention, making it difficult for a child to do well in school and in social situations.

A syndrome usually characterized by inattention, hyperactivity, and impulsive behavior, ADHD is a close relative to attention deficit disorder (ADD), which affects the attention and impulse control of individuals but is not characterized by hyperactive behavior. Both syndromes run in families, and boys with ADHD tend to outnumber girls by at least 3 to 1.

For people with ADHD, life is like a fast-moving carousel where sounds, smells, sights, and thoughts are constantly stopping and starting, or even spinning out of control. Although many children seem to outgrow the disorder, at least 30 percent are affected throughout adulthood. However, many adults with the disorder remain unaware that they have it unless one of their children is diagnosed with ADHD. These adults may simply think of themselves as disorganized and unable to stay on task; they may consequently suffer in both personal relationships and careers as a result.

ADHD is a disorder that may require a combination of behavioral counseling, special education, nutritional intervention, and medications over many years. In the last decade, scientists have learned a great deal about the disorder and are now in the process of pinpointing its biological basis—a process certain to lead us to more effective preventive strategies and treatments.

No single cause has yet been identified for ADHD. In fact, ADHD will probably one day prove to be an umbrella term for a number of associated disorders. However, researchers around the world have come a long way in identifying environmental and biochemical links to the disease, and in tracking just how the disorder affects the brain's metabolism and function.

Leading investigators are currently exploring the association between ADHD and factors such as genetic influences, prenatal alcohol consumption, environmental toxins, brain damage, food allergies, fatty acid deficiency, faulty glucose metabolism in the brain, and thyroid abnormalities. All these studies promise us a better understanding of the syndrome, based on what we are rapidly learning about how ADHD affects the brain's biochemistry.

Although clinicians currently differ on the best treatment for ADHD, all agree that a multimodal approach—one that incorporates dietary measures, counseling, special academic strategies, and possibly medication—is best.

In this chapter, we present ADHD from the onset of symptoms to diagnosis, discussing the full range of treatments based on what we know today about the syndrome's impact on the brain's biochemistry. Finally, we offer an aggressive treatment plan incorporating the most current studies available on nutritional therapies and medications.

## What Goes Wrong in ADHD, and Why?

Research concerning the possible causes of ADHD revolves around this key concept: Our ability to pay attention is an active process, not a passive one.

In order to selectively sort out stimuli from our environment— as a child must do in a classroom, or a manager must accomplish at work—certain brain regions must kick into gear while others are inhibited. In other words, the act of paying attention requires the integrated input and coordination of several brain regions.

The most important of these is the tiny brain stem area known as the "locus ceruleus." This brain region is responsible for sending messages to the front of the brain to alert us to the tasks at hand.

In essence, you can't pay attention if you aren't awake, and the brain's locus ceruleus acts as a coach on the sidelines, yelling at his players on the field to rally together. The chemical messenger that the locus ceruleus relies on most to send those messages is norepinephrine, the "revving up" neurotransmitter. Two things have to happen for proper signaling: the levels of norepinephrine must be finely regulated, and the receptors for that neurotransmitter must be ready to receive messages.

If the locus ceruleus is damaged—through injury, stroke, or infection—higher brain systems receive inadequate signals and lose track of what's happening on the playing field. A number of studies worldwide have demonstrated that damage to the brain regions that control our ability to pay attention produces symptoms of impulsiveness, compulsivity, and short attention span.

While there is no structural derangement of these important brain regions in people with ADHD, scientists are now unearthing clues that point to functional derangements of these same brain structures. One of the most important tools used in recent years to perform those studies is PET scanning, a sophisticated radiological device that measures brain metabolism.

Quite simply, when your brain is at work, its cells demand glucose as a primary energy source. PET scans allow scientists to measure brain activity by determining the amount of glucose being used by certain brain regions. As you would expect, areas of high glucose metabolism show that the brain is working harder, which lowered glucose demands are equated with diminished brain metabolism. These PET scans actually produce visual images of brains at work.

In examining the brains of people with ADHD, scientists have used PET scans to demonstrate that certain areas of their brains show a decreased use of glucose and diminished brain metabolism. The results were not a surprise: People with ADHD suffer most from impaired glucose use and lowered activity in those areas of the brain controlling our ability to pay attention.

Currently, scientists are striving to determine the genetic, prenatal, physical, and biochemical factors that may lead to decreased glucose metabolism in people with ADHD. They are also searching for other differences between people with the disorder and those who are not affected. Soon, we hope to have new protocols for treating ADHD that may successfully increase activity in the parts of the brain so crucial to our ability to pay attention.

## •*A Genetic Predisposition*

In diagnosing ADHD in you or your child, a health care practitioner should take a complete family history to determine whether any other members in the family show signs of being affected by the disorder. This is because ADHD and other attention disorders run in families. Children diagnosed with ADHD generally have at least one close relative with ADHD, the majority of identical twins share the trait, and about a third of all fathers who had ADHD as children go on to bear children with the disorder. Scientists are currently tracking a gene that may be the culprit involved in transmitting ADHD in some families.

## •*Fetal Alcohol Syndrome and ADHD*

Research on the brains of developing fetuses have offered scientists a number of clues about neurological disorders. A human brain begins its growth from a few cells and develops into a complex, three-pound organ comprised of a billion specialized cells. Now, research reveals that mothers who indulge in heavy alcohol consumption during pregnancy put their unborn infants at risk for fetal alcohol syndrome (FAS), a disorder characterized in children by low birth weight, an impaired intellect, and certain physical defects. Children born with FAS often show the same hyperactivity, low impulse control, and inability to pay attention as those children who are diagnosed with ADHD.

## •*Lead Exposure May Impair Brain Development*

According to the *Cecil Textbook of Medicine,* we are all lead poisoned. Our current lead burden is about 200 times greater than what it was in preindustrial times, and that exposure can have disastrous effects on the brain.

Lead is found in dust, soil, and flaking paint in areas where leaded paint and gasoline were once used, and is even in some of our drinking water pipes. Sadly, over 400,000 U.S. babies are diagnosed with toxic blood lead levels annually.

We have known for some time that lead is toxic enough to lead to miscarriage or brain damage, as it interferes with normal brain development and function by accumulating in the mitochondria of brain cells, causing them to swell and perform abnormally.

Other studies have revealed that chronic lead poisoning can cause problems in the digestive tract and nervous system. Now, researchers tracking behavioral symptoms in young children who show evidence of lead poisoning have discovered that those symptoms include irritability, sleep disturbances, difficulties concentrating, motor incoordination, and symptoms of ADHD.

A number of recent studies support the argument that children who suffer from overexposure to lead are at risk for ADHD. For example, when researchers at the University of Massachusetts School of Public Health evaluated the relationship between lead levels and ADHD by testing for this toxic metal in the tissues of children via hair analysis, they found a striking correlation between ADHD and high lead levels.

In addition, New York researchers from a number of institutions collaborated in comparing the blood and urine lead levels of hyperactive children to those of youngsters who showed no signs of hyperactivity. They found a clear association between hyperactivity and raised lead levels.

Further studies have demonstrated that children with the highest level of lead in their bones are more likely to suffer from behavioral problems and attention disorders. In an investigation performed at the University of Pittsburgh School of Medicine, researchers discovered that many of the children tested who showed high bone lead levels were also diagnosed with ADHD— although these children actually had normal blood lead levels.

Since even low levels of lead exposure are associated with hyperactivity, attention deficit disorder and development failure, the American Academy of Child and Adolescent Psychiatry recommends that any child with behavioral disorders or learning disabilities be tested for lead exposure.

In addition, as you will see in our "Complete Blueprint for Care" section of this chapter, clinicians are now exploring ways to help mend lead-induced, impaired brain function with nutritional agents such as zinc and NAC. These supplements have proven beneficial in alleviating lead toxicity and the symptoms of ADHD.

Additionally, dietary deficiencies of calcium, iron, and zinc can enhance the negative effects of lead on cognitive and behavioral development by increasing lead absorption and not being able to compete for lead in many biochemical processes in the body.

### • The Relationship Between Thyroid Dysfunction and ADHD

Your thyroid gland is located at the base of your neck and, appropriately enough, wraps around your windpipe and is shaped like a bow tie.

This important gland produces hormones with a profound impact on brain and body metabolism because they regulate the rates at which various cells consume oxygen. One of those hormones is thyroxine, which regulates the pace of chemical activity in your body. In other words, the more thyroxine you have in your bloodstream, the more chemical reactions occur.

A variety of recent observations has now led investigators to conclude that a relationship exists between thyroid dysfunction and ADHD. For instance, up to 70 percent of all children with a condition known as "generalized thyroid resistance" to thyroid hormones also demonstrate ADHD symptoms.

Thyroid resistance refers to the decreased ability of body tissues to respond to those important pace-setting thyroid hormones. Patients with thyroid resistance suffer from altered glucose uptake by cells—a feature that we now know impairs brain metabolism. Altered glucose uptake is linked to ADHD if that diminished brain activity happens to be in the brain regions responsible for our ability to pay attention and control our behavior.

In addition, thyroid hormones are important in regulating the "coaching" neurotransmitter, norepinephrine. That's because thyroid hormone augments the ability of brain cell receptors to bind with norepinephrine, promoting the effect of that neurotransmitter on neurons (see below).

### •What Causes Impaired Thyroid Function and ADHD?

Scientists are currently investigating possible reasons for impaired thyroid function and the subsequent inability of the locus ceruleus to produce appropriate levels of norepinephrine.

Synthetic chemicals like PCBs, phenols, thiols, and excessive histamines are possibly at fault. According to recent investigations, these environmental toxins can lead to thyroid dysfunction and brain damage, especially in the attention-governing region of the locus ceruleus.

As we mentioned earlier, thyroid hormones help regulate body chemistry by assisting neurotransmitters in their mission to attach to cell membrane receptors. Remember that, when a neurotransmitter like norepinephrine attaches to a membrane receptor, it causes a particular chain of chemical reactions in that cell. So, it is only logical that anything that interferes with that crucial neurotransmitter binding process is going to alter brain chemistry.

Now, animal studies have demonstrated that certain toxins may actually block normal thyroid hormone action because they successfully mimic the hormones and are transported to brain cells in their stead. For example, mice fed low doses of PCBs develop a "spinning syndrome" which causes them to circle their cage incessantly, and the most common neurological damage found in lab animals exposed to PCBs early in life is hyperactivity.

Our brain cells are primed to receive hormonal messages— so much so that they readily accept synthetic imposters in their stead. Luckily, our bodies have devised an elaborate detoxification mechanism to cleanse the body of these interfering imposters. This mechanism, which we call "methylation," depends largely on a powerful enzyme known as SAM (s-adenosyl methionine), which studies now show to be an effective nutritional supplement in treating adults with ADD.

## •Fatty Acids, Thyroid Function, and ADHD

As you already know, the brain is composed mostly of fats. Up to 25 percent of the brain's white matter consists of phospholipids derived from essential fatty acids, which play an important role in forming cell membranes. Fatty acids are also essential precursors to making the substances that brain cells use to communicate with one another.

Clinicians have associated fatty acid deficiency with a variety of skin problems and increased allergies—symptoms that typically affect hyperactive children. Now, a number of studies have gone one step further to identify an essential fatty acid deficiency in many hyperactive children. For example, a 1995 study published in *The American Journal of Clinical Nutrition* showed a correlation between low omega-3 blood levels and ADHD in young boys.

Why should a fatty acid deficiency lead to thyroid dysfunction and ADHD?

As you learned earlier, when a neurotransmitter binds to its cell membrane receptor, it triggers the formation of second messengers responsible for translating the event into a proper cellular response. Essential fatty acids act as these second messengers. They belong to a family of chemical compounds known as "eicosanoids," which are necessary for cell-to-cell communication by receiving the neurotransmitter's signal and ensuring that the next chemical step takes place inside the brain cell. Therefore, a deficiency in fatty acids can lead to inappropriate neurotransmitter effects and altered brain chemistry.

In particular, essential fatty acids play a role in maintaining normal sleep-wake cycles and in stimulating the growth of myelin, the insulating substance on nerve cell fibers that makes better electrical communication possible. Later on in this chapter, we will offer specific recomendations for adding fatty acids to the diet to ease the symptoms of ADHD.

## •Dietary Factors: Food Additives, Allergies, and Sugar

In 1973, Dr. Benjamin Feingold first proposed that artificial flavors and artificial colors cause hyperactivity. These include benzoic acid, BHA, BHT, MSG, butylene glycol, potassium bisulfate, potassium and sodium nitrate, sulfites, tartrazines, dyes, and flavorings. In addition, Feingold recommended that hyperactive children avoid salicylates, derivatives of salicylic acid, which is commonly used as a preservative or in the manufacture of aspirin. In addition, salicylates are found in almonds, apples, cherries, pickles, grapes, raisins, oranges, peaches, plums, strawberries, tomatoes, vinegar, and phenolic compounds added to foods.

In a 1994 study at the North Shore Hospital-Cornell Medical Center, researchers Boris and Mandel discovered that eliminating reactive foods—those foods apt to cause a reaction in a sensitive individual—and artificial colors from the diet may actually be of benefit in treating some children with ADHD. This is only one of many such studies equating food additives with increased irritability, restlessness, sleep disturbances, and other negative behaviors among people with ADHD.

Another study, this one published in *Pediatrics,* also reported on sugar as a possible instigator of aggressive behavior, hyperactivity, and attention problems exhibited by children with ADHD. In that investigation, children with ADHD who consumed large amounts of sugar showed greater inattention in performing tasks. However, they demonstrated no more aggressive behavior than usual.

Meanwhile, investigators reporting in *The Journal of Autism and Developmental Disorders* revealed that children with ADHD experienced abnormal rhythms in the stress hormone cortisol—an abnormality frequently associated with problems in metabolizing carbohydrates. Yale researchers have confirmed that children with ADD may have a problem in metabolizing glucose, in that offering children doses of oral glucose significantly diminished their ability to concentrate.

While conflicting data exists regarding food allergies, sugar, and ADHD, clinicians generally recommmend modifying the diet to eliminate possible allergenic foods, dietary chemical preservatives, and sugar to determine whether a particular individual with ADHD or ADD is affected by any of those factors. We will discuss this procedure in greater detail below.

## TABLE **7**

### WHAT CAUSES ADHD?

1. A genetic predisposition.

2. Overexposure to lead, PCBs, or other environmental toxins.

3. Mother's prenatal cocaine or alcohol consumption, especially if fetal alcohol syndrome is also present.

4. Brain damage by physical trauma before, after, or during birth.

5. Thyroid dysfunction.

6. Fatty acid deficiency.

7. Faulty glucose metabolism in certain brain areas that regulate the ability to pay attention.

8. Food allergies and an inability to process refined sugars.

### • *Why Are More Boys Affected with ADHD than Girls?*

As we mentioned earlier, the key neurotransmitter involved in coaching the brain to pay attention is norepinephrine. Inadequate norepinephrine levels may result in the inattentiveness experienced by people with either ADD or ADHD. The hyperactivity component of ADHD—which is evidenced by far more boys than girls—is most likely related to inappropriate levels of another neurotransmitter we have discussed earlier in this book: dopamine. Girls may be more likely to have ADD instead of ADHD because estrogen inhibits the reception of dopamine by neurons.

# A Complete Blueprint for Care

## When Should You Suspect ADHD or ADD?

Like so many neurological illnesses, attention disorders such as ADD and ADHD offer no clear physical symptoms that can be clearly determined through x-rays or blood tests. In general, clinicians must examine a wide range of characteristic behaviors over a period of time in order to diagnose ADD or ADHD. Professionals will determine whether these behaviors are excessive, have lasted a long time, and are a continuous problem rather than a temporary response to surroundings or stimuli.

In general, people with ADHD are diagnosed on the basis of these three characteristic behaviors:

### •Hyperactivity

The person with ADHD will always be in motion. Unable to remain at rest for long periods of time, these individuals bounce and twitch in their seats, touch everything, and noisily tap their pens or chew their fingernails. They often try to do several things at once, as they are unable to focus on just one. People with ADD do not exhibit this hyperactive behavior.

### •Poor Impulse Control

People with either ADD or ADHD are likely to find it impossible to stop themselves from blurting out inappropriate statements or responding immediately to stimuli. Children with ADHD or ADD are apt to sock a child in anger, for example, and are oblivious to dangers inherent in their actions. These children might jump from high places or cross the street without looking, for example, because they fail to stop and think about possible outcomes.

### •Inability to Pay Attention

Everyone daydreams, and most small children have trouble paying attention for long stretches at a time. However, people who are inattentive as a result of ADD or ADHD truly cannot keep their minds on any one thing and find it difficult to pay attention long enough to learn something new. They are easily distracted by irrelevant sights and sounds, fail to pay attention to details, and find it difficult to follow instructions or keep track of personal belongings.

# Diagnosing ADHD/ADD: Ensure the Right Diagnosis

A number of specialists are qualified to diagnose ADHD. These include psychiatrists, psychologists, family physicians, pediatricians, and neurologists. The specialist will begin by gathering information as a way of ruling out other possible causes for the individual's inattention and behavior at home, at school, and at work.

Monitoring tools for ADHD/ADD include the Conners Teacher/Parents Rating Scales, ADD-H Comprehensive Teacher Rating Scale, Child Attention Problems Rating Scale, Yale Children's Inventory, DSM-III-R, Wechsler Intelligence Scales for Children, Child Behavior Checklist, Attention Battery, Test of Variables of Attention, the Wide Range Achievement Test, Developmental Test of Visual Motor Integration, and the Learning Efficiency Test II.

Basically, ensuring the right diagnosis means ruling out the following possible causes for inattention, poor impulse control, or hyperactivity:

## • Childhood Depression

Symptoms of childhood depression can also include irritability, poor concentration, and acting-out behavior, all of which may be inappropriately attributed to ADHD. A qualified health care professional should evaluate the child for depression as well as ADHD.

## • Petit Mal Seizures

Symptoms of petit mal seizures include frequent staring episodes, which may be misinterpreted as poor concentration and hyperactivity. Petit mal seizures may also be associated with eye-blinking movements. Diagnosing petit mal seizures requires an EEG.

## • Lead Toxicity

Clinical lead poisoning has been associated with an increased incidence of hyperactivity in children. It is important to test children exhibiting hyperactivity for lead toxicity, although lead toxicity alone is generally not the only cause of ADHD.

### • Thyroid Abnormalities

Any routine diagnostic workup should include routine measurements of thyroid and thyroid antibodies. The presence of thyroid antibodies may be caused by "autoimmune thyroiditis," a syndrome which may lead to hypothyroidism. Furthermore, as we have seen here, certain chemicals may take over thyroid hormone receptor sites and subsequently impair thyroid function. Abnormal thyroid tests should, of course, be evaluated by a qualified physician.

## The First Step to Take: Rule Out Food Allergies

Eliminating the possibility of food allergies is key in establishing a healthy diet for individuals with attention disorders, as a number of food items may exacerbate symptoms in a small percentage of individuals. While food allergy tests can measure antibody levels and diagnose food allergies, most individuals can employ simple elimination diets without the risk of obtaining the false results common to some food allergy tests.

In simplest terms, you can begin an elimination diet by avoiding the most common allergenic foods for several days. These include milk, wheat, yeast, citrus, egg, chocolate, soy, corn, sugar, and the food additives and salicylates we listed above. Following this initial cleansing, your clinician can monitor behavioral and symptomatic responses as a single, potentially offending food is brought back into the diet at a time.

Although eliminating food allergies this way involves significant initial dietary modifications, this is the most cost-effective, efficient way to detect allergies. In one study conducted at the Institute of Child Health in London, for instance, using an elimination diet resulted in significantly improving the behavior of a group of hyperactive children. Their behavior worsened when they were challenged with allergy-provoking foods.

Similarly, in the prestigious medical journal *Lancet,* investigators reporting on a study with 185 hyperactive children on an elimination diet supported the concept that food allergies are associated with hyperactivity.

We recommend that all individuals considering this method of testing for food allergies do so under the guidance of a qualified nutritionist or physician.

## The Second Step to Take: Explore the Role of Sugar in Causing Hyperactivity

As you already know, foods high in refined sugar are the major culprits responsible for poor eating habits leading to nutritional deficiencies. In addition, because of the potential relationship between refined sugar intake and abnormal cortisol rhythms among individuals with ADHD, and because of the impaired brain glucose metabolism found in many people with ADHD, we recommend assessing the patient with ADHD for both reactivity to sugar intake and potential glucose intolerance.

### •Don't Overlook the Possibility of High Lead Levels

Given that so many studies have correlated the incidence of high lead levels with attention disorders, behavioral problems, and learning disabilities, your health care practitioner will no doubt question you about prenatal lead exposure and request the results of all lead tests. Most often, testing for lead is done through blood serum and urine; however, studies are currently underway to determine whether hair analysis is a viable alternative.

If testing confirms lead poisoning, your clinician may advise you to consider chelation therapy under a specialist's care. Chelation involves administering an agent that binds to the metal and promotes its excretion through the urine. However, although this type of therapy may possibly be valuable in treating lead poisoning in individuals with ADHD, it has potentially severe adverse effects and requires close monitoring, especially of kidney function.

In general, lead poisoning is promoted by zinc, calcium, and iron deficiencies. Therefore, a good route for parents concerned about lead toxicity may be to ensure that children are receiving adequate zinc, calcium, and iron (see below).

## Nutritional Therapies You Should Consider Now

In addition to adopting the two-step healthy diet guidelines for healthy individuals we outline in *The Brain Wellness Plan,* individuals with ADHD should modify their diets according to the outcomes of food allergy elimination diets and assessment for both a reactivity to refined sugar and glucose intolerance.

### • Add Chromium, Zinc, and the Complete B-Complex to Improve Glucose Metabolism

Individuals who demonstrate glucose intolerance should incorporate fully reacted chromium and zinc chelates and the complete B-complex vitamins into their diets. Chromium is essential for maintaining normal glucose control, while zinc and the B vitamins assist in the utilization of insulin and glucose.

*RECOMMENDED DAILY DOSES WITH FOOD:*

| | |
|---|---|
| Chelated zinc | 15 mg (children 6–12); 30 mg (adult) |
| Chelated chromium | 100 mcg (children 6–12); 300 mcg (adult) |
| B-complex vitamins | As found in any children or adult multivitamin-mineral supplement |

Look for fully reacted mineral chelates, as these are the best absorbed and utilized.

### • Use Fatty Acids to Improve Brain Metabolism

Throughout this book, we have illustrated the importance of omega-3 and other essential fatty acids in building up cell membranes and improving their fluidity. In addition, essential fatty acids are necessary ingredients for the body to make prostaglandins and create myelin sheaths around nerve fibers, the white matter that facilitates cell-to-cell communication.

Independent investigators around the world have reached the conclusion that a deficiency in fatty acids may therefore adversely affect behavior, as a result of lowered prostaglandin production and poor communication between brain cells.

With respect to ADHD, a number of studies confirm the importance of fatty acids in improving the brain metabolism of children. For example, when Purdue University researchers studied the significance of fatty acids in metabolism among subjects with ADHD, they made a startling discovery: These people suffered from significantly lower plasma concentrations of the two most important fatty acids, EPA (eicosapentaenoic acid) and DHA (docosahexaenoic acid).

In another study, a subgroup of ADHD subjects with EFA deficiency symptoms demonstrated significantly lower DHA levels in plasma as compared to ADHD subjects who showed no deficiency in essential fatty acids. Investigators concluded that decreased cellular concentrations of DHA can adversely affect behavior by possibly decreasing the production of prostaglandins that act as modulators of nerve transmission, and believe that the cerebral cortex's proper function may be negatively affected since DHA is the predominant polyunsaturated fatty acid in that part of the brain.

Finally, animal studies have demonstrated that animals restricted to diets low in omega-3 fats have impaired behavioral and neurological functions.

We urge all individuals with attention disorders to consider being tested for fatty acid levels, and to boost fatty acid intake through a combination of DHA, fish oil omega-3 fats, and flaxseed oil. (Flaxseed oil contains linolenic acid, a precursor to the omega-3 fats.)

**RECOMMENDED DAILY DOSES WITH FOOD:**

DHA                100 mg (children 6–12) 300 mg (adult)

(Look for the trademarked Neuromins™
from Martek Biosciences Corporation.)

Max EPA™    1–2 g (children) 3 g (adult)
Flaxseed oil  1 tbsp for children and adults
          (organic, cold pressed, keep refrigerated)
Vitamin E   100 IU (children 6–12) 400 IU (adult)

All these fatty acid boosters should be taken with meals.

### •*Keep Up Zinc Levels to Improve ADHD Symptoms*

As we have seen in previous chapters, zinc plays a number of important roles in keeping you healthy—particularly when it comes to maintaining a vital immune system.

Now, as scientists continue to map out the various ways in which zinc is needed by your body, a number of studies are pointing to an association between zinc deficiency and ADHD. One such 1996 study, published in the *Journal of Child Psychology and Psychiatry,* revealed a statistically significant correlation between zinc and fatty acids, in that both were decreased in children with ADHD.

In another study, this one conducted at Ohio State University, investigators found a relationship between zinc deficiency and response to stimulant therapy among people with ADHD. (Stimulants such as Ritalin are commonly used to treat children with ADHD, as you will see in our section on medications.) Basically, this study showed that children diagnosed with ADHD may be zinc deficient, and that this deficiency may result in their poor response to stimulant therapy.

Investigators are now exploring the connection between associated deficiencies in zinc and fatty acid levels. The most likely explanation for the association is that zinc is necessary for the body to produce the enzyme which converts precursor (''parent'') fat compounds into the essential fatty acid DHA.

Based on these results, we suggest that every individual diagnosed with ADHD be tested for a zinc deficiency. In the event that a zinc supplement proves necessary, we recommend a fully reacted zinc chelate.

RECOMMENDED DOSE: 15 mg for children (6–12) and 30 mg for adults, with a meal. Look for a fully reacted zinc chelate.

### •Amino Acids: Of Controversial Benefit

Over the past ten years, a number of investigators have been examining the benefits of using the amino acids tyrosine and phenylalanine for treating ADHD. Interest in these amino acids stems from the association of ADHD with deficiencies in norepinephrine or dopamine. Researchers at Ohio State University, for example, have studied plasma amino acids in ADHD patients and found that these individuals had significantly lower levels of several, including tyrosine and tryptophan. These scientists concluded that a general deficit in amino acid transport, absorption, or both may lead to ADHD symptoms.

Since tyrosine and phenylalanine have been shown to increase catecholamine synthesis, scientists have reasoned that the therapeutic application of those amino acids might have positive effects. Unfortunately, several studies have reported no benefits in supplementing the diets of patients with ADHD with either amino acid. Further investigation into this area is ongoing.

## Other Neuroimmunomodulating Substances to Discuss with Your Health Care Practitioner

### • SAM: Improve the Brain's Housekeeping Ability

The brain requires a continuous recycling of neurotransmitters. For a neurotransmitter to produce its desired effect, it can exist in its active form for only a very short time. It is then broken down by the brain, so that by-products can be recycled for future use in building fresh neurotransmitter messengers.

The brain recycles stale neurotransmitter by-products through two distinct detoxification mechanisms which we call "transulfation" and "transmethylation." As you can probably guess, "trans" means "transfer," and in this case the brain is transferring either a sulfur compound of a methyl compound out of the brain.

Why is is necessary for the brain to transfer these compounds anywhere? Because those forms are easier for the kidneys and liver to dispose of than the more complex compounds.

One key substance involved in transulfation is SAM (s-adenosyl methionine). Ths hearty, high-energy compound helps break old neurotransmitters into compounds that can more easily be excreted from the body.

Researchers have discovered that increased levels of SAM can significantly enhance the body's ability to detoxify itself of various substances, including old neurotransmitters. SAM is currently under study as a potential therapeutic agent in ADHD as a result.

For instance, in a trial completed by researchers in Israel, adults diagnosed with ADHD took oral doses of SAM and found that their symptoms improved significantly. Another study conducted by researchers at the University of California at Los Angeles revealed that 75 percent of adults diagnosed with ADHD reported feeling calmer, more in control, and slowed down enough to be more productive after taking SAM.

Based on these and similar studies supporting the use of therapeutic SAM in treating ADHD, investigators believe that SAM may actually help mop up old neurotransmitter materials and improve the way fresh neurotransmitters bind to cell membranes.

While the mechanisms by which SAM may benefit people with ADHD are still unclear, we suggest discussing the possibility of taking SAM supplements with your healthcare practitioner.

> **RECOMMENDED DOSE:** Consult with your health care practitioner about sources and dosages. We recommend that adults take 400 mg tablets, without exceeding 2400 mg per day. Children should be administered half that amount.

## Medications Used to Treat ADHD

In most cases, medications are used as a last resort in treating the symptoms of ADHD, particularly in children. However, there are a number of medications on the market that are considered effective. We have listed those that are most commonly prescribed.

## • *Clonidine*

If we prescribe any medication at all for a child diagnosed with ADHD, it is usually clonidine. Clonidine is actually a medication used for blood pressure, and acts on the receptors of the brain stem that receive dopamine and norepinephrine, the two neurotransmitters responsible for your ability to pay attention and monitor your own impulsive behavior. We typically do not prescribe Clonidine for children under five, as major side effects may include fatigue and hypotension.

## • *Ritalin*

By far the most commonly prescribed medication of ADHD, Ritalin is a stimulant that treats only the symptoms of ADHD without addressing the underlying disease process. Furthermore, despite its wide use, Ritalin has become a subject of controversy in the past decade because of its potential side effects, including insomnia, diminished appetite, and the appearance of motor tics. We recommend Ritalin in only the most extreme cases of ADHD, and as a last resort.

## • *Effexor (venlafaxine)*

A newly developed antidepressant, venlafaxine has been shown to be successful in treating some adults with ADHD. This medication appears to enhance neurotransmitter activity in the brain, and is a potent inhibitor of both norepinephrine and serotonin reuptake, which means more of these neurotransmitters are left around for the benefit of cell use.

## • *Piracetam*

Originally introduced as a memory-enhancing medication, Piracetam improves the metabolism of brain cells through various mechanisms. Animal studies have shown that Piracetam has the potential to enhance learning and memory, and this medication is currently being investigated for its potential in treating neurological illnesses as wide-ranging as Alzheimer's and ADHD.

In adults with attention disorders, some clinicians are now

prescribing Piracetam to enhance attention. The drug has no appreciable effect on hyperactivity, and its effect on children has not been fully studied.

## Putting It All Together

We were as determined as Clarissa to use medication as a last resort in treating her son Jon for ADHD. Instead, we began by referring the family to a nutritionist, who helped them eliminate allergies to certain foods and food additives and coached them in finding ways to improve Jon's eating habits. The elimination diet showed that Jon suffered from a significant milk allergy. Additional testing proved that Jon showed no evidence of abnormal glucose intolerance.

We immediately suggested that Jon discontinue drinking milk, and Clarissa began including juices and other nonmilk drinks in Jon's lunchbox for school. In addition, we added supplements of 400 mg of DHA, 3 g of fish oil, and 2 tablespoons of flaxseed oil to boost Jon's essential fatty acid intake and improve his brain metabolism, as Jon suffered from the excessive thirst and dry skin common to so many children with ADHD who are deficient in omega-3 fatty acids. We also recommended that Jon be given 15 mg daily of zinc, and assessed Jon for adequate calcium and iron intake as we offered suggestions for good dietary sources.

Clarissa and Ray began seeing a family counselor with Jon to learn how to better moderate their son's behavior, and worked closely with Jon's preschool and kindergarten teachers to assess his progress and adjust his learning environment where needed. Today, Jon is in the first grade, reads well, and is well liked by his classmates. Although he is still a highly energetic boy, he suffers none of the frustration in the classroom that he experienced in his early years, and is much more manageable to home.

Now that you have an overview of attention disorders and of how they may impact on brain metabolism, you are probably eager to begin investigating a complete ADHD treatment protocol for yourself or someone you love. We encourage all patients with ADHD to seek individual and family counseling to help resolve behavioral and emotional issues, and to investigate the educational support available through public and private schools.

## Dietary Protocol

- Use elimination diets under the guidance of a professional to assess allergies to foods and food additives, and to evaluate the effect of sugar intake.
- Assess for adequate calcium and iron intake. If deficiencies exist, add 1000 mg of calcium, 400 mg of magnesium, and 15 mg of iron (use fully reacted mineral chelates).
- In the presence of glucose intolerance, add 200 mcg of fully reacted, chelated chromium taken twice daily.

*Daily Nutritional Supplements*

| | |
|---|---|
| DHA (look for the preferred Neuromins™) | 300 mg (adult), 100 mg (children) |
| Fish oil (look for MaxEPA™) | 3 g (adult), 1–2 g (children) |
| Flaxseed oil (cold-pressed, organic, keep refrigerated) | 1 tbsp |
| Chelated zinc | 15 mg (children, 6–12); 30 mg (adult) |
| Vitamin E | 400 IU (adult), 100 IU (children) |

All supplements are to be taken with food.

*Other Neuroimmunomodulating Substances to Discuss with Your Health Care Practitioner*

SAM (s-adenosyl methionine)

*Medications*

Clonidine
Ritalin
Effexor (venlafaxine)
Piracetam

# CHAPTER 10

# CHRONIC FATIGUE SYNDROME

Alicia was thirty-seven when she came down with a particularly severe flu. She had always been able to kick that sort of thing within a few days, but this time was different. Although she stayed in bed for more than a week and her fever and headache did seem to ease a bit, she just couldn't seem to get enough rest to feel like herself again.

Admittedly, Alicia's job as a social worker left her feeling burned out—there were always too many clients and not enough time in the day to see them all—but something was definitely wrong with her. Even the simplest things, such as carrying the laundry downstairs, left her completely fatigued.

Weeks turned into months, and yet Alicia wasn't getting any better, despite the fact that her family physician had found nothing wrong. She was having trouble concentrating at work, she wasn't sleeping well, her lymph nodes felt swollen from time to time, and her headaches and fevers continued. Her husband was losing patience with her, and told her to "get a grip" on herself because he wasn't about to be married to someone who made him fetch and carry for her every day.

Finally, Alicia began seeing a round of specialists. A psychologist suggested depression, while an infectious disease specialist tested her for all sorts of illnesses she had never even heard of before. It was a full year, in fact, before a neurologist confirmed Alicia's diagnosis: She was suffering from chronic fatigue syndrome.

"Is this ever going to get better?" she pleaded. "I feel like I'm on death's door."


## Chronic Fatigue Syndrome: An Overview

Chronic fatigue syndrome (CFS) began drawing the national spotlight in 1985, when Nevada physicians reported an unusually high number of unrelated patients suffering from disturbingly similar symptoms. Those symptoms included chronic fatigue, headaches, fevers, and aching muscles. The Centers for Disease Control recognized the condition and dubbed it "chronic fatigue syndrome" for its one common symptom—the debilitating exhaustion that affects everyone with CFS.

Today, interest in CFS has prompted investigators around the world to scrutinize its causes and pathways. What should be clearly stated at the outset of any discussion of CFS is this: Although up to a quarter of all U.S. adults attending primary care clinics report that fatigue is a major problem affecting their lives, the fatigue that serves as the hallmark symptom of CFS is much more persistent and severe.

Accompanying symptoms of CFS vary according to the individual, and may cover everything from joint pain to fevers, and decreased memory capability to depression. Because of this, a CFS diagnosis is usually made on the basis of symptoms lasting at least six months and only after eliminating other possible conditions that could be causing the fatigue and other symptoms described.

In fact, one of the biggest problems associated with the disease is lack of credibility—patients suffering from CFS have been accused by friends and coworkers of being hypochondriacs or of having "that yuppie flu." And despite the fact that an illness resembling CFS was described by an English physician, Sir Richard Manningham, as early as the mid-1700s, even some physicians refuse to be convinced that the condition is real. Patients often have to see several physicians, including specialists in neurology, immunology, and psychiatry before being successfully diagnosed—a process that is as frustrating as it is wearing.

To date, scientists have not yet uncovered the cause of CFS.

Most potulate that it is due to a combination of multiple factors acting together rather than the result of a single cause. The one common factor many patients report is the onset of a severe illness, such as bronchitis, gastrointestinal illness, sore throats, or hepatitis, just before developing CFS.

CFS is not a fatal disease, but at its most severe can be debilitating enough to impair an individual's ability to work, care for a household, or otherwise enjoy life. Although about 70 percent of the people diagnosed with CFS are young white women in the middle class, this disparate proportion may have to do with the fact that women are more apt to seek out medical care than men, or because the skepticism surrounding this diagnosis prevents individuals from other groups from seeking help.

Although neither cause nor cure has yet been discovered for this complex syndrome, our evolving biochemical knowledge about brain and immune system functions has brought us much closer to finding effective treatments for CFS.

In this chapter, we explore the most current theories developed to explain how CFS affects the brain and the immune system. We will then describe the disease in detail from onset to diagnosis, and present an aggressive treatment plan based on today's scientific findings in nutrition, neurology, and immunology.

## What Goes Wrong in Chronic Fatigue Syndrome, and Why?

Researchers at top medical centers around the world are conducting basic research and clinical studies to determine just what causes CFS.

To date, investigators have uncovered clues leading us to believe that (1) chronic fatigue syndrome may be an example of the hypothalamus failing to properly regulate the brain's influence on the immune system; (2) a clear relationship exists between CFS and one type of hypotension; (3) the symptoms of CFS may be produced, at least in part, by inadequate muscle metabolism of oxygen and nutrients; and (4) CFS may be due to an immune disorder.

## • The Brain's Master Conductor Misses a Beat

From our earlier chapters on the brain-immune connection, you know that the hypothalamus is the key intersection for communication between your body's brain and immune system. Now, scientists believe that hypothalamic dysfunction may be at the root of CFS.

The tiny, pea-sized hypothalamus coordinates the activity of the brain and immune system by regulating the messenger molecules that travel between the two. In this way, the hypothalamus is the central control tower when it comes to coordinating the immune system; the endocrine system, which consists of the hormone-producing endocrine glands; and the autonomic nervous system, which regulates cardiac or smooth muscle cells and glands.

Among the most important glands to be under the control of your hypothalamus are the adrenal glands—small, triangular organs, one on top of each kidney. Although no more than a few centimeters in size, these glands are responsible for synthesizing some of your body's most essential hormones, including cortisol.

The hypothalamus produces a messenger hormone known as corticotropin-releasing hormone, or CRH, which is sent out by the brain as a chemical messenger to provoke the necessary responses among all three body systems mentioned above. CRH is especially critical for coordinating your body's response to stress because it provokes your adrenal glands to make cortisol.

Many people diagnosed with CFS suffer from low levels of CRH. Since that hormone is so essential in gearing up the adrenal glands to secrete cortisol, many people with CFS suffer from impaired adrenal gland function during times of infection or other types of stress. In other words, CFS is a state of relative adrenal insufficiency which occurs as a result of reduced CRH levels and, consequently, a reduced ability to manufacture cortisol. According to studies done at the National Institute of Mental Health and other research centers, cortisol is a necessary part of the body's defense against stressors such as toxins and infections. The low levels of CRH and, consequently, of cortisol could cause many of the common symptoms of CFS, such as fatigue, swollen lymph nodes, muscle and joint pain, insomnia, and depression.

As you will see later in this chapter, one of the revolutionary new treatments for people with CFS involves nutritionally supporting adrenal gland function as a way of restoring a healthy brain-immune connection.

## •Hypotension and CFS: Why Do These Two So Often Go Together?

Recently, a landmark study performed at Johns Hopkins University proved that many people with CFS are also afflicted with a syndrome known as "neurally mediated hypotension" (NMH).

Just what is NMH? Under normal circumstances, your body is able to maintain a steady blood pressure and pulse while you change positions—from lying down to getting to your feet, for example. However, in NMH, the body has lost this ability to regulate the effects of heart rate and blood pressure during postural changes. This causes the blood pressure to decrease so much that, when the patient changes position, the result may be severe fatigue or headaches because of reduced blood flow to the brain.

NMH is typically diagnosed through a "tilt test," in which the patient lies on a table that the physician tilts in different directions, all the while monitoring the effects those position changes have on blood pressure and pulse. The Johns Hopkins study revealed that the majority of patients diagnosed with CFS also suffer precipitous falls in their blood pressure or heart rates during such tilt tests, indicating that they have NMH, too.

Why would CFS and hypotension go hand-in-hand so often?

Again, the answer boils down to having inadequate levels of CRH.

The autonomic nervous system is responsible for regulating the functions of cardiac and other smooth muscle cells in the body. One particular component of this system, the "sympathetic nervous system," specifically controls pulse and blood pressure.

As with the adrenal glands, the CRH hormone is the brain's lead messenger in regulating the sympathetic nervous system. If the brain is not producing enough of this hormone, it's like pressing the accelerator in a car that has run out of gas: there just isn't enough CRH to do the job. Consequently, the body is unable to maintain a steady blood pressure level or pulse rate.

The reasons for such a CRH deficiency are still under speculation. One possible explanation is that there has been a disruption in the normal feedback loop between the brain, the immune system, and the endocrine system, possibly owing to an infection or environmental toxin.

### • Oxidative Muscle Metabolism: Not Enough Cellular Energy for Muscles

Many patients with CFS complain that they are so tired that they feel as if they are dragging about with their feet encased in heavy boots. Exercise may further aggravate their symptoms of fatigue and muscle pain.

Studies conducted with CFS patients performing heavy exercise have shown that these individuals exhibit higher heart rates than people without the disorder and are unable to fully activate skeletal muscles during intense fatigue. In addition, researchers have found abnormalities in the mitochondria of muscle cells—the tiny energy factory organelles responsible for cellular metabolism—among people with CFS.

At the Medical College of Pennsylvania, for example, investigators have studied people with CFS to see if the ability of their muscle cells to metabolize oxygen and other nutrients to produce energy in the form of ATP (adenosine phosphate) is affected by their condition.

They found that this ability was significantly reduced, and concluded that patients with CFS are affected by a functional abnormality in "oxidative muscle metabolism," or the way their muscle cells burn oxygen and other nutrients to produce energy. In our "Complete Blueprint for Care" section, you will discover that one particular nutritional supplement, coenzyme Q10, can help boost the ability of muscles to perform work among patients with CFS.

## • What About Immune System Complications Owing to Epstein-Barr Virus and Other Viral Complications?

Early research indicated that some CFS patients had unusually high levels of antibodies to Epstein-Barr virus (EBV), the virus that causes infectious mononucleosis. Typically, acute illness eventually subsides in people infected with EBV, with the virus remaining dormant. However, in some CFS patients the antibody levels remained high, suggesting to some investigators that CFS might be a sort of chronic EBV.

Now, new evidence reveals that many other individuals without CFS also have high EBV antibody levels, leading most scientists to now conclude that EBV does not lead to CFS in most patients. However, recent studies do support the concept that EBV and a number of other viruses may be reactivated in patients with CFS, though whether this viral reactivation causes CFS or is a result of the syndrome remains to be seen.

Scientists are continuing to investigate the link between CFS and immune system complications that occur as a result of viral infections. Studies reveal that patients with CFS may have low levels of white blood cell activity, for example, or an abnormal distribution of white blood cells. Among those investigating the link between CFS and immune system breakdowns are researchers at the University of Miami School of Medicine. They have found that cytokines such as certain interleukins and tumor necrosis factor are elevated in patients with CFS, indicating that these patients suffer from the same sort of overzealous immune system activity prominent in so many other neurological illnesses.

Overall, then, in treating CFS, it is essential to ensure that patients receive the proper nutrition to build a healthy immune system.

# A Complete Blueprint for Care

Although there is no cure for CFS, you can take aggressive steps now toward (1) adjusting your lifestyle to better manage the condition, (2) enhancing your brain's production of the essential hormone CRH; (3) addressing the possible connection

TABLE **8**

## WHAT CAUSES CHRONIC FATIGUE SYNDROME?

- The hypothalamus produces inadequate levels of CRH (corticotropin-releasing hormone), which leads to a subsequent breakdown in adrenal gland production of cortisol.

- An association between neurally mediated hypotension and CFS.

- Insufficient energy metabolism by muscle cells.

- Immune system complications provoked by prior viral infections.

between hypotension and CFS; (4) boosting muscle metabolism; and (5) building back your immune system.

## When Should You Suspect CFS?

CFS is often difficult to diagnose because individuals with the disorder vary widely in their symptoms, from being severely disabled and even bedridden to simply being unusually fatigued following stressful events. To add to the mysterious nature of this disorder, symptoms tend to come and go over time. CFS is often diagnosed only after many months and after other secondary causes of fatigue have been ruled out.

Generally, CFS is diagnosed according to these core criteria:

- Clinically evaluated, unexplained persistent or relapsing chronic fatigue that is not the result of ongoing exertion or alleviated by rest; this fatigue often results in an impaired ability to keep up with one's work, education, and social and personal life;
- The presence of four or more of the symptoms listed below, all of which must have lasted or recurred during at least six consecutive months since the fatigue first set in:
  - sleep disturbances
  - tender lymph nodes

- sore throat
- short-term memory loss
- muscle pain
- joint swelling
- headaches

## Secondary Causes of Fatigue to Be Ruled Out During Diagnosis

For a certain CFS diagnosis, it is first essential to rule out other possible causes of the pervasive fatigue experienced by patients, such as:

### •Lyme Disease and Other Chronic Infections

A tick-borne illness characterized by rash and arthritis, Lyme disease is currently endemic to several areas of the United States. Two of the most frequent symptoms of Lyme disease are fatigue and malaise; in fact, estimates are that up to 80 percent of patients with Lyme disease experience significant and long-term fatigue.

Other infections that can cause fatigue include HIV, hepatitis, and chronic yeast infections. All these chronic infections can be ruled out through laboratory blood tests or spinal fluid analysis.

### •Thyroid Disease

Hypothyroidism or low levels of circulating thyroid hormone characteristically produce fatigue and other associated symptoms, including constipation, slowed thinking, and excessively dry skin. Hypothyroidism can be ruled out through an analysis of thyroid-stimulating hormone (TSH) by ultrasensitive assay.

### •Vitamin Deficiencies

A number of different vitamin deficiencies, especially low levels of B12, are characterized by lassitude and fatigue. Again, the possibility of these deficiencies should be ruled out through laboratory tests in diagnosing CFS.

*• Neurally Mediated Hypotension*

Although NMH does not cause CFS, it may be useful for patients experiencing headaches and lightheadedness to have a "tilt test" to determine if NMH is causing those symptoms. As we discussed earlier, many patients with CFS also have NMH.

## The First Step to Take in Treating CFS: Lifestyle Adjustments

Patients with CFS must take good care of themselves through adjusting their work or personal habits to minimize stress, improve sleep habits, and eat according to *The Brain Wellness Plan* guidelines for nutrition set out earlier in this book. The truth is, although this disease can be long-term and debilitating in some, many people do recover from CFS or manage the symptoms very well over time.

## Dietary Suggestions You Can Incorporate Now

The nutritional therapy for CFS gives considerable attention to eliminating food allergies, enhancing immune and adrenal function, supporting the production of energy by muscle cells, addressing debilitating symptoms, and correcting nutritional deficiencies that might otherwise hamper rehabilitation.

Patients with CFS commonly experience gastrointestinal symptoms such as flatulence and poor digestive function. The "friendly bacteria" we describe in *The Brain Wellness Plan*, along with the other nutrients listed there that specifically support gastrointestinal functions, should help alleviate those symptoms.

*• See a Qualified Nutritionist to Evaluate Individual Dietary Restrictions*

Patients with CFS should seek the care of a qualified nutritionist to assess nutritional deficiencies and diagnose food allergies. In many cases, nutritionists treating CFS will advise an elimination diet, whereby all possible allergenic foods are avoided for a period of time and then reincorporated gradually to assess for food allergies.

The nutritionist will also evaluate whether the patient has a sugar intolerance, which would warrant a higher protein, moderate carbohydrate diet taken in small, frequent meals throughout the day.

## Nutritional Supplements to Begin Taking Now

### • Boost Adrenal Function through Nutrients and Herbs

The symptoms associated with low adrenal function include excessive fatigue, weakness, depression, insomnia, swollen lymph nodes, allergies, and headaches—a list of symptoms strikingly similar to the symptoms for CFS.

As we have noted earlier, people with CFS are often suffering from insufficient levels of adrenal hormones such as cortisol, owing to low levels of corticotropin-releasing hormone (CRH) and subsequently impaired adrenal gland function.

The adrenal glands contain the highest concentrations of vitamin C in the body, and vitamin C is an essential cofactor in the enzyme precursor to making norepinephrine, the neurotransmitter which plays the largest role in regulating our sympathetic and parasympathetic nervous system. Therefore, it is essential that people with CFS limit adrenal gland stressors such as sugar and caffeine and incorporate the nutrients necessary for optimal adrenal support. These include vitamin C, zinc, vitamin B6, pantothenic acid, and magnesium. These nutrients all play necessary roles in the manufacture of hormones by the adrenal glands.

For instance, a recent study published in *Lancet* revealed that patients with CFS have lower red cell magnesium and showed that magnesium supplements led to improved energy, better emotional states, and less pain among those patients.

Herbs have also proven beneficial in supporting the adrenal

glands. For example, animal studies have shown that one of the best nutrients for supporting everything from enhancing adrenal gland hormone production to inhibiting adrenal atrophy is ginseng. The active ingredients in ginseng responsible for boosting adrenal function are "ginsenosides" in Panax ginseng extract and "eleutherosides" in Siberian ginseng; both have proven effective in promoting hormone production in the adrenal glands.

Another herb useful in managing CFS is standardized licorice extract (although this should be avoided if hypertension or depression is present). The ingredient in licorice that has proven active in affecting adrenal function is called "glycyrrhizin." Glycyrrhizin acts by stimulating the adrenal glands to produce cortisol and to prolong cortisol action. One 1995 article, published in the *New Zealand Medical Journal,* described the use of licorice in treating CFS and concluded that licorice upped cortisol production.

**RECOMMENDED DAILY DOSES:**

| | |
|---|---|
| Vitamin C | 4 g, in divided doses. The use of calcium ascorbate may help prevent GI tract upset. |
| Pantothenic acid | 50 mg |
| Zinc | 30 mg (Use a fully reacted mineral chelate for efficient absorption and utilization.) |
| Magnesium | 600 mg in divided doses. (Use a fully reacted mineral chelate for efficient absorption and utilization.) |
| Ginseng | 500 mg standardized Panax ginseng or Siberian ginseng |
| Licorice | 150 mg standardized extract, as long as no hypertension or depression is present |

All these nutritional supplements should be taken with meals.

## • Enhance Muscle Metabolism

As we described earlier, many patients with CFS suffer from impaired energy metabolism in their muscle cells. In addition to the full B-complex vitamins we recommend in *The Brain Wellness Plan*, we suggest that all patients with CFS incorporate coenzyme Q10 and creatine to enhance muscle metabolism by assisting the production of ATP in muscle cells.

If you recall, ATP (adenosine triphosphate) is the energy currency of cells, serving as the chemical intermediate through which at least half of the energy of cells is released during the breakdown of carbohydrates, fats, and proteins. Half of the energy produced goes to the cell, while the other half is released as heat energy.

One of the most essential cellular ingredients for producing ATP is coenzyme Q10. And as an antioxidant, coenzyme Q10 helps protect the cell from free radical damage.

Creatine phosphate is just as essential to energy production in muscle cells, because ATP cannot be produced unless creatine phosphate is around to donate a phosphorus molecule. A nutrient naturally found in our bodies, creatine is made from the amino acids aginine, methionine, and glycine. It has been shown to increase muscle mass through promoting better protein synthesis within muscle fibers, and is essential for muscle contractions.

Researchers from the Queen's Medical Center in the United Kingdom established the important role of creatine in ATP muscle production. In addition, they have shown that supplemental creatine can significantly enhance muscle strength and reduce the amount of ATP lost during exercise.

We recommend that all patients with CFS incorporate a supplement of coenzyme Q10, and add creatine supplements if engaged in regular exercise.

**RECOMMENDED DAILY DOSES:**

| | |
|---|---|
| Coenzyme Q10 | 200 mg, with food |
| Creatine monohydrate | 5 g, on an empty stomach (Use only if involved in a regular exercise regime.) |

## • *Rebuild Your Immune System Through General Multivitamin and Antioxidant Supplements*

Because so many patients with CFS also have weakened immune systems, our ''Complete Blueprint for Care'' emphasizes supporting immune function through nutrients and herbs with proven roles as immune boosters.

Research in recent years has shown that a number of nutritional substances have the power to enhance the immune system. Studies have revealed the following:

- Reduced zinc levels are associated with decreased white blood cell activity.
- Vitamin A maintains the integrity of the immune system by stimulating and enhancing white blood cell activity and antibody response.
- Deficiencies in B vitamins can reduce antibodies and cell-mediated immune responses.
- Vitamin D can function as a steroid hormone, in that a number of white blood cells possess receptors for active vitamin D and are regulated by this vitamin.
- Selenium deficiency inhibits macrophage activity and the production of the tumor necrosis factor cytokine.
- Copper deficiency impairs macrophage function, the production of white blood cells, and healthy cytokine response;
- Vitamin C can modulate immune response by activating white blood cells and enhancing cytokine production.
- A deficiency in coenzyme Q10 is associated with viral infections.
- Vitamin E (tocopherols and tocotrienols) serve as antioxidants with immune-related functions, in that they can lower prostaglandin E2 levels and enhance immunity.

In general, all of the above nutrients are easy to come by, provided that patients with CFS follow our recommendations in Chapters 3 and 4 of *The Brain Wellness Plan.*

## • Enhance Glutathione Levels to Further Protect Cells from Free Radicals

Free radical damage to DNA, proteins, and fats in cells is a major contributor to degenerative diseases such as CFS. In addition to the free radical damage done to cells during normal cellular metabolism, immune cell activity, and other processes, patients with CFS are also more vulnerable to damage by free radicals produced by external factors such as fatty foods, radiation, and cigarette smoke.

During any challenge to the immune system—as in CFS—additional antioxidants are required to help scavenge the free radicals produced as a result of immune system battles. The antioxidant complex described above will certainly help ameliorate any antioxidant deficiency. However, because patients with CFS are particularly vulnerable to fatigue, headaches, fevers, muscle pain, and other stresses on the immune system, we also recommend that these individuals boost their glutathione levels as extra insurance against free radical oxidation injury.

The ability of cells to maintain an adequate glutathione status is critical to our health. Additionally, through the activation of the enzyme glutathione transferase, glutathione inactivates toxic compounds that may hinder immune response.

The best strategy for boosting cellular glutathione levels is through supplements of NAC (n-acetyl-cysteine), lipoic acid, and selenium, which is an essential ingredient in making the glutathione transferase enzyme.

**RECOMMENDED DAILY DOSES:**

| | |
|---|---|
| Lipoic acid | 200 mg, with food |
| NAC | 1 g, on an empty stomach |
| Selenium | 200 mcg, with food (Do not exceed this amount.) |

## • Polyphenols: Strong Antioxidants to the Rescue

Polyphenols are strong antioxidants with a number of other important functions. For example, polyphenols can attach themselves to certain pro-oxidant metals, such as iron, thereby reducing the capacity of that metal to produce free radicals in the body. In addition, polyphenols can inhibit the effects of toxic arachidonic acid in the body by inhibiting lipoxygenase, the enzyme that converts arachidonic acid into leukotrienes (mediators of allergies and inflammation). Finally, polyphenols can gear up the immune system to combat viral infections.

One supplement of particular benefit in treating CFS is Pycnogenol®, a derivative extract from the bark of a French marine pine tree which contains a number of important polyphenolic components. As a dietary supplement, it acts as both an antioxidant and an immune system booster.

Animal studies conducted at the University of Arizona showed that Pycnogenol® has the power to maintain healthy immune system function by restoring cytokine imbalances and increasing white blood cell activity.

Our food supply is filled with polyphenols. Excellent sources include red wine, green tea, berries and other fruits, soybeans, and dark vegetables. The best supplement sources include Pycnogenol®, rhododendron extract, grape seed extract, pine bark extract, and herbs such as bilberry, ginkgo, and milk thistle.

---

**RECOMMENDED DAILY DOSES:** The best supplement sources include Pycnogenol®, fruit polyphenols, grape seed extract, pine bark extract, and herbs such as bilberry, ginkgo, and milk thistle. Choose one of the excellent sources of polyphenols listed below or look for a formula that combines several sources.

| | |
|---|---|
| Pycnogenol® or pine bark extract | 120 mg, with a meal |
| Grape seed extract | 120 mg, with a meal |
| Fruit polyphenols | 120 mg, with a meal |

---

### • Use Essential Fats to Strengthen Cells

Supplementing the diet of individuals suffering from immune-related disorders has proven that omega-3 fats such as EPA (eicosapentaenoic acid) and DHA (docosahexaenoic acid) can have a profound role in diminishing unwanted inflammation and building up immune function.

Omega-3 fatty acids from fish and algae sources can successfully compete with omega-6 fatty acids from corn and other vegetable oils, which can positively influence immune system function, as omega-6 fats have been shown to heighten inflammatory responses while suppressing the immune system.

In 1994, an article published in *Medical Hypotheses* demonstrated that offering supplements of omega-3 fats and gamma-linoleic acid (GLA) from primrose or borage oil significantly improved the immune systems of patients with CFS participating in the study. Scientists in other investigations have shown that omega-3 supplements can help reduce cytokine-mediated inflammation.

Food sources for omega-3 fats include fatty fish (salmon, mackerel, herring, and tuna). The omega-3 fatty acids can be easily obtained by using any of the following supplements: flaxseed oil, MaxEPA™ brand of fish oils, and the vegetarian source of DHA (look for the trademarked Neuromins™ brand). We also suggest adding primrose or borage oil.

**RECOMMENDED DAILY DOSES:**

| | |
|---|---|
| MaxEPA™ | 2 g |
| DHA (Neuromins™) | 300 mg |
| Primrose or borage oil | 2 g |

These supplements should all be taken with meals.

## •Add These Herbs to Stimulate Your Immune System

Any immune nutritional protocol should include the following herbs for optimum support:

**Astragalus membranaceous:** 500 mg standardized extract daily. May be used long-term. Enhances antibody response, increases helper T-lymphocytes and natural killer cell activity, and promotes production of certain cytokines.

**Echinacea:** 250 mg standardized extract daily. Use for seven to ten days with three-week rest intervals. Stimulates macrophages, enhances white blood cells, and cytokine production.

**Reishi mushroom:** 4 g standardized extract daily. Increases production of cytokines and natural killer cells, boosts white blood cell activity. May be used long-term.

**Shiitake mushroom:** 4 g standardized extract daily. Stimulates white blood cell and natural killer cell activity, activates macrophages and promotes their recognition of antigens, and boosts white blood cell proliferation. May be used long-term.

**Maitake mushroom:** 4 g standardized extract daily. Activates macrophages, natural killer cells, and white blood cells. Also stimulates cytokine production. May be used long-term.

## What Other Neuroimmunomodulators Should You Discuss with Your Health Care Practitioner?

### • If the Tilt Test Reveals NMH, Consider Salt and Fludrocortisone

As so many patients with CFS also are diagnosed with NMH (neurally mediated hypotension), we advise our patients to have a tilt test. If the tilt test proves positive for NMH, we recommend increased salt intake or a mineral corticoid drug, Fludrocortisone, to reestablish your body's ability to maintain a steady blood pressure and pulse. Salt and Fludrocortisone do this by helping the kidneys to retain sodium and, therefore, to retain body fluids and maintain blood pressure.

### • Address Sleep Disorders with Melatonin or Medication

Fatigue is the hallmark of CFS. Yet despite how tired they are, many patients with CFS report that they have difficulty getting to sleep and that their sleep is often disturbed. Whether CFS promotes sleep disturbances or sleep disturbances are simply a significant contributor to the overwhelming fatigue experienced by patients with the disorder, a health care practitioner should certainly thoroughly evaluate sleep patterns in treating patients with the disorder.

If sleep disturbances are reported, we recommend that patients try melatonin first to help restore normal sleep patterns. If that fails, there are a number of other herbs and medications that have proven beneficial in helping patients with CFS normalize sleep-wake cycles. Consult with your health care practitioner to find the proper type of sleeping aid and correct dosage.

### • Improve Hypothalamus Function through SSRIs like Zoloft, Paxil, or Prozac

As we discussed at the outset of this chapter, one of the newest theories posed to explain CFS involves hypothalamic dysfunction. In treating patients, we often prescribe medications such as Zoloft, Paxil, or Prozac, as these SSRIs (selective serotonin reuptake inhibitors) have the ability to restore any abnormalities in serotonin receptors located in the hypothalamus.

As you may recall, the serotonin neurotransmitter plays a leading role in regulating sleep, appetite, sexual behavior, mood swings, the cardiovascular system, and immune system activity. Serotonin imbalances in the brain have been linked to a wide range of neurological disorders, including autism and depression.

Among its other features, serotonin is able to restore the activity of CRH, one of the body's most influential hormones. In a significant number of patients with CFS, SSRIs have demonstrated the ability to raise brain serotonin levels and reset CRH activity, therefore leading to healthier adrenal gland function.

## Putting It All Together

In putting Alicia back on the road to good health, we encouraged her to take a close look at the long hours she was keeping in her position as a head social worker at a busy urban clinic. Alicia subsequently cut her hours in half and began taking a yoga class in the evenings.

Taking melatonin supplements restored Alicia's ability to get a good night's sleep, and she worked closely with a nutritionist to evaluate her eating habits and reduce her sugar intake. In addition, we referred Alicia to a medical center for a tilt test to rule out the possibility of NMH.

To support Alicia's flagging adrenal glands and immune system, we added all the nutritional supplements described in the protocol below. A month later, we estimated that Alicia had improved about 40 percent in most of her symptoms. She was less tired, experienced fewer headaches and fevers, and seemed to have a much higher energy level.

However, as Alicia still had relapses now and then, suffering occasional fevers and headaches during bouts of fatigue that caused her to cut back on her daily activities still further, we prescribed Zoloft. Now, more than two years later, Alicia has improved by more than 75 percent in all the symptoms she reported. She has been able to add a moderate exercise program and has returned to working full-time.


With this overview of chronic fatigue syndrome, you are probably anxious to begin—or to help someone you love get started—investigating the ways in which you can boost your immune function, muscle metabolism, and adrenal function through an aggressive protocol.

Here is our summary guideline for treatment.

| | |
|---|---|
| *Dietary Modifications* | Follow *The Brain Wellness Plan.* |

*Daily Nutritional Supplements*

| | |
|---|---|
| Vitamin C | 4 g in divided doses with food. The use of calcium ascorbate may help prevent GI tract upset. |
| Pantothenic acid | 50 mg |
| Zinc* | 30 mg of zinc glycinate or zinc histidinate with food |
| Magnesium* | 600 mg of magnesium glycinate or magnesium citrate, taken in divided doses with food. |
| Licorice | 150 mg of standardized extract, as long as no hypertension or depression is present |

| Coenzyme Q10 | 200 mg with a meal |
| Creatine monohydrate | 5 g on an empty stomach (use only if involved in a regular exercise program) |
| Lipoic acid | 200 mg with a meal |
| NAC (n-acetyl-cysteine) | 1 g on an empty stomach |
| Selenium | 200 mcg with a meal (Do not exceed this amount.) |

Choose one:

| Pycnogenol R | 120 mg, with a meal |
| Fruit polyphenols | 120 mg, with a meal |
| Grape seed extract | 120 mg, with a meal |
| MaxEPA™ | 2 g with a meal |
| DHA (Neuromins™) | 300 mg with a meal |
| Primrose or borage oil | 2 g, with a meal |

*To Stimulate Immune Function*

| Astragalus membranaceus | 500 mg of standardized extract |
| Echinacea | 250 mg of standardized extract (Use for seven to ten days with three-week stop intervals.) |
| Reishi mushroom | 4 g of standardized extract |
| Shiitake mushroom | 4 g of standardized extract |
| Maitake mushroom | 4 g of standardized extract |
| Ginseng | 500 mg of standardized Panax ginseng or Siberian ginseng |

Look for fully reacted mineral chelates for efficient absorption and utilization.

*Additional Neuroimmunomodulators to Consider*

Salt or Fludrocortisone
Melatonin

*Medications*

Medications to restore sleep patterns
Selective serotonin reuptake inhibitors (Prozac, Zoloft, Paxil, etc.)

# CHAPTER 11

# DEPRESSION

Despite her status as a star basketball player and senior class president, eighteen-year-old Doreen began suffering from mild episodes of depression. Generally, she worked her way through her infrequent "blue periods," as she called them, by forcing herself to continue to keep up with schoolwork even if she holed up at home and watched television for hours on end instead of socializing.

By the time Doreen was a junior in college, however, her episodes of depression had become frequent enough to interfere with her natural zest for life. She gradually lost interest in both sports and academics, and she dropped off the basketball team and began missing classes. Her appetite faltered and she began losing weight. Some mornings, she was too tired to drag herself out of bed, and when she did, she seldom bothered to dress. What was the point, when she didn't feel like going anywhere or seeing anyone?

Doreen tried using the college counseling service and was referred to a social worker, who attempted to address the source of her depression through therapy. However, Doreen could think of nothing to say that would shed any light on her mood.

"I feel so numb, I just can't enjoy things anymore," she confessed. "I feel hopeless all the time. And yet, someone looking at my life from the outside would say I have nothing to complain about."

The social worker recognized that Doreen was suffering from depression, and referred her to a psychiatrist, who suggested that Doreen continue her therapy once a week and try a prescription for antidepressants. While Doreen wanted to continue the therapy, she was resistant to the idea of medication. She sought help at our office because she was looking for an alternative solution.

"I just don't like the idea of medication," Doreen explained. "I'm the sort of person that doesn't even take aspirin for a headache. Isn't there something else I can try?"

## Depression: An Overview

If you or someone you love is suffering from depression, rest assured that you are not alone. At present, one in twenty Americans suffers from clinical depression and requires medical treatment, and one person out of every five will suffer a depressive episode at some point. These statistics boost depression to the top of all public health problems in this country.

Abraham Lincoln suffered from depression most of his adult life. So did many famous musicians, writers, and artists including Peter Tchaikovsky, Robert Schumann, Gustav Mahler, Hans Christian Anderson, Ernest Hemingway, Charles Dickens, Isak Dinesen, Mary Shelley, Virginia Woolf, Buonarroti Michelangelo, and Paul Gauguin.

Yet, it is only in recent decades that depression has truly become understood for what it really is: a chronic disease of the brain that is completely different from the sort of mental anguish that follows loss, or the "down" cycles in life's ups and downs.

The risk for depression runs in families. However, many people are diagnosed with clinical depression who have no family history of the disease at all. Although people over sixty-five are four times more likely to suffer from depression than those in other age groups, children and teenagers can suffer from the disease, too. Currently, experts estimate that at least 5 percent of all adolescents suffer from depression. More than twice as many women are currently being treated for depression as men; however, this may be due to men denying that they need treatment. Almost two-thirds of the people who have one depressive episode will go on to have at least four more in their lifetime.

Where has research brought us so far in understanding this pervasive disease?

Scientists have at last succeeded in building a bridge between depression and brain mechanisms. Through two decades of research, we have come to understand that depression is closely linked to the dysfunction of two neurotransmitters in the brain, particularly serotonin. The diverse treatments that have emerged to treat depression as a result of this research—including monoamine oxidase inhibitors, tricyclic antidepressants, and SSRIs—have been devloped on the basis of this research.

About two-thirds of all people diagnosed with clinical depression readily respond to treatment with short-term therapy combined with an antidepressant. People who do not respond to the first antidepressant prescribed will most likely respond to another, and symptoms of depression will ease within a few weeks' time as a result.

Tragically, however, many people with depression fail to find help in time. About fifteen percent of people with this disorder commit suicide as a result.

In this chapter, you will discover just what research has taught us about the ways in which depression alters brain function and metabolism, particularly in the relationship between the hypothalamus and the rest of the body.

More exciting still, you will learn how sophisticated studies in neurology and nutrition have contributed to our ability to prescribe a power-packed treatment plan to prevent and treat depression. This plan adds the latest breakthrough nutritional and hormonal therapies to our existing strategies of using therapy and antidepressants.

## What Goes Wrong in Depression, and Why?

In recent decades, a number of interesting scientific studies have begun to describe just what happens in the brain to affect the mood disorders characterizing clinical depression.

The most important of these findings include (1) the possibility that depression is an inherited disease, (2) the relationship between fatty acids and depression, (3) the breakdown in the hypothalamus's ability to regulate the production of an important hormone called CRH, and (4) the ways in which reduced brain levels of the norepinephrine and serotonin neurotransmitters alter brain chemistry and cause depression.

### • For Some, Depression May Be in the Genes

Clinical studies conducted over the past decade have offered persuasive evidence that the risk for severe depression runs in families and is most likely genetic. Just as researchers have mined human chromosomes to determine how diseases such as Parkinson's and Alzheimer's are transmitted in families, so are a number of scientists at prestigious medical centers now racing to discover how gene mutations might account for depression.

However, clarifying just which genes are responsible for this debilitating illness is extremely complicated. For one thing, depression is so common in our population that scientists speculate the disorder must be due to several different gene mutations rather than just one.

And unlike the degenerative disorders we can describe according to the clear changes in brain structure they provoke, depression is variable in its pathways. This makes it much more difficult to track, both in individuals and in groups.

### • A Deficiency in Omega-3 Fatty Acids: Weakened Cells Contribute to the Altered Brain Chemistry that Heralds Depression

Now, various studies have demonstrated that lowering plasma cholesterol through diet and medication may indeed be healthier for our hearts—but has the unwanted side effect of increasing episodes of depression and suicide.

For example, in the famous Framingham Study, the largest ever to examine the relationship between lowered cholesterol and decreased heart disease, researchers made this disconcerting discovery: People participating in the study who lowered their cholesterol did, in fact, suffer less from heart disease. However, more of the study's participants committed suicide compared to the rest of the population.

Yet other studies have shown that societies apt to consume large amounts of fish—which contain high amounts of omega-3 fatty acids—have lower cholesterol levels than other populations as well as a lower incidence of heart disease—*without* raising rates of depression.

Where does the discrepancy lie between our population and theirs? What are we doing wrong?

Researchers now believe that the answer lies in the types of fatty acids we consume. Over the past two decades, Americans have bought into the idea that eating margarine and corn oil can save our lives by lowering our cholesterol and preventing heart disease. Unfortunately, we have replaced saturated fat with too many omega-6 unsaturated fats, rather than the omega-3 unsaturated fats that are so essential to brain health.

Like all cells in your body, your brain cells are surrounded by membranes composed chiefly of fats (also called phospholipids). The basic function of those membranes is to regulate the way that biological substances travel in and out of cells.

A saturated fat when incorporated in a cell membrane differs considerably in structure and function from unsaturated fat in a cell membrane. Furthermore, as you learned from our general description of fatty acids in the general nutrition chapters of *The Brain Wellness Plan*, there are different types of polyunsaturated fats. The two broad groups are the omega-3 and omega-6 fatty acids.

Today, science supports the view that decreasing your intake of omega-3 fatty acids may impair brain function, increase your risk of heart disease, and raise your risk of suffering from depression. In other words, these essential fatty acids are vital to both your physical and psychological health.

Recently, as reported in the *American Journal of Clinical Nutrition,* scientists have shown that the omega-3 fatty acid phosphatidylserine (PS) increased dopamine, norepinephrine, and epinephrine concentrations in animals.

In another multicenter study conducted with 404 elderly patients, adminstering 300 mg of PS caused them to become less depressed. Studies like these have led many clinicians around the world to conclude that adequate omega-3 fatty acid intake may be essential in preventing and treating depression.

From all of this, we can conclude that omega-3 fatty acids are essential for all aspects of healthy brain cell metabolism. This is because the brain requires specific fatty acids to synthesize hormones, cell membranes, and components of the immune system.

If your diet is composed mostly of saturated fats (animal fats) and deficient in unsaturated fatty acids, the result is that your brain cell membranes will become less fluid—which can have a devastating effect on the way that neurotransmitters bind to their receptors.

But it's not enough simply to seek out unsaturated fatty acids; they have to be the right kind. The omega-3 unsaturated fatty acids are required to ensure healthy interactions between neurotransmitters and their receptors. A deficiency in omega-3 fatty acids results in the reduced ability of a neurotransmitter to bind to its receptor. Thus, omega-3 fatty acid deficiency is linked to depression, because the neurotransmitters we rely on to safeguard against depression—namely, norepinephrine and serotonin—cannot properly bind to their receptors and perform their function within the brain.

As part of our "Complete Blueprint for Care" in this chapter, we will show you just how you can help prevent and treat depression by raising your intake of essential omega-3 fatty acids.

## •Inadequate Tryptophan May Lead to Low Brain Serotonin Levels . . . and Depression

The theory that low levels of serotonin in the brain may lead to clinical depression has been supported by numerous clinical studies examining the spinal fluid and brain tissue of people who died as a result of depression, usually by suicide. Those investigations have shown that these individuals did, indeed, have low levels of brain serotonin.

As we have already discussed, low levels of omega-3 fatty acids may impair the way serotonin binds to receptors on cell membranes. Now, new evidence has shown that reduced serotonin activity may also be the result of low levels of its essential chemical precursor, tryptophan. Individuals with depression have much lower tryptophan blood concentrations in relation to other amino acids than do people without the disorder.

Studies have shown that reducing the intake of dietary tryptophan can induce depression in some people, as there is simply not enough of this valuable ingredient to make the serotonin needed. In addition, tryptophan can be broken down by the liver before it's ever made into serotonin.

Interestingly, depressed patients often have an elevated cortisol level, as you will see in the discussion below, which in turn induces the activity of a certain liver enzyme capable of dismantling tryptophan. When the liver breaks down more tryptophan, less is around to act as a precursor to serotonin, and low levels of serotonin are clearly associated with depression. Because of the adverse effect of cortisol on the synthesis of serotonin from tryptophan, administering doses of tryptophan alone may prove to be an ineffectual treatment for depression.

In fact, using tryptophan as an antidepressant either by itself or with traditional antidepressant therapy has not demonstrated significant benefits; it may even have severe adverse effects if tryptophan is combined with any of the selective serotonin reuptake inhibitors (SSRIs) such as Prozac or Zoloft. That's because the combination of this nutrient with SSRIs may actually lead to the production of too much serotonin in the brain—a potentially life-threatening condition.

## • A Faulty Hypothalamus Communication Loop May Lead to Depression

The hypothalamus is a tiny, pea-sized brain organ that serves as a sort of United Nations for important meetings between various body systems. The body systems that rely on the hypothalamus to orchestrate communication speak via chemical molecular messengers. They include the immune system; the endocrine system, which is made up of all hormone-producing glands; and the autonomic nervous system, which is responsible for monitoring cardiac and other smooth muscle functions.

As in so many neurological illnesses, depression can result when this miniature organ fails to orchestrate effective chemical communication. Over half of all patients diagnosed with severe depression exhibit striking abnormalities in brain metabolism that centers right in the hypothalamus. One of the most devastating consequences of this hypothalamic breakdown is that patients with depression experience a marked increase in the release of corticotropin-releasing hormone, or CRH.

What causes the hypothalamus to ratchet up CRH production when it shouldn't? And why should an abundance of this natural hormone lead to depression?

The mechanisms of the hypothalamic breakdown are still being explored. To date, we only know that the hypothalamus becomes overstimulated and sends too much CRH to your adrenal glands. These two small, triangular organs, which are just a few centimeters in size and located on top of your kidneys, respond to the frantic signaling by the hypothalamus in the only way they know how: they produce an overabundance of cortisol, your body's stress hormone.

As blood levels of cortisol rise in patients with depression, tryptophan production dips down and, consequently, leads to a reduced availability of that essential serotonin ingredient. The brain can then no longer make enough serotonin to go around. This leads to a Catch-22 situation, in that adequate brain serotonin is required to turn down the hypothalamus and slow down its production of CRH.

The different classes of antidepressants used to treat depression today all seem to work by increasing levels of serotonin, norepinephrine, and dopamine in the brain. Although we do not yet fully grasp just how increasing the concentrations of these neurotransmitters alleviates depression, most likely these medications change the way that the brain's cell membranes bind with these essential mood-altering neurotransmitters.

## • What About the Relationship Between Vitamin Deficiencies and Depression?

In *The British Journal of Psychiatry* and other journals, scientists have reviewed the relationship between a number of vitamin

TABLE **9**

## WHAT CAUSES DEPRESSION?

- A genetic predisposition.

- Faulty neurotransmitter function owing to weakened brain cell membranes and impaired neuron receptor binding.

- Low levels of tryptophan, serotonin's key precursor.

- Overproduction of cortiocotropin-releasing hormone by the hypothalamus, causing the adrenal glands to produce too much cortisol.

- Vitamin deficiencies, which may cause depressive symptoms.

deficiencies and depressive states. Essentially, scientists have linked depression to deficiencies of riboflavin (B2), pyridoxine (B6), folic acid, and vitamin C.

This was not really a surprise, since the classical symptoms of these vitamin deficiencies mimic those of clinical depression. At Harvard Medical School's MacLean Geriatric Hospital, both geriatric and young adult depressive subjects were found to be deficient in B2, B6, and B12. Their data supports the hypothesis that poor nutritional status, especially in certain B vitamins, can contribute to depression.

In addition, several studies have demonstrated that impaired folic acid metabolism and folic acid deficiency are present in many patients diagnosed with depression. This may be because a folic acid deficiency impairs your body's ability to synthesize BH4, a cofactor essential for the body to make dopamine and serotonin. SAM, which acts as an antidepressant, is also dependent on folic acid for its metabolism.

# A Complete Blueprint For Care

As we have seen, the symptoms which doctors and therapists use to diagnose depression are linked to alterations in brain chemistry. Nobody knows exactly what event acts as a catalyst for the changes in brain metabolism in any one individual, as the disease varies so much in its pathways. Depression can be the result of hormonal changes, chemical effects owing to other chronic illnesses, spontaneous changes in chemistry, psychological triggers, or some combination of these factors.

Sometimes, this metabolic alteration returns to normal after a few years, even without medical treatment. Better still, up to 80 percent of all individuals diagnosed with clinical depression are readily treatable within a few weeks of diagnosis through a combination of therapy and antidepressant medications. In addition, revolutionary insights into the power of nutrients to boost brain health and mend faulty neurotransmitter synthesis and binding have led us to recommend aggressive nutritional therapies to restore healthy chemical balances in the brain.

## When Should You Suspect Depression?

Everyone feels sad from time to time. So how do you determine if you're suffering from the "blues" or true, clinical depression?

Basically, in clinical depression, feelings are out of proportion to any external causes. In addition to feeling sad, depressed individuals may experience a numb or empty feeling and a noticeable loss in the ability to take pleasure in life. Depression is a disease of the brain, but it ends up as a "whole body" illness affecting they way you eat, sleep, and think. It is not a passing mood, and people with depression cannot simply pull themselves up by the bootstraps, keep their chin up, or put the best face on the situation. When it comes to depression, none of these clichés holds true.

The DSM-III-R, the official diagnostic and statistical manual for psychiatric illnesses, defines the most common types of depression according to these criteria:

• *Major Depression*

Major depression causes people who suffer from it to cease functioning normally. Treatments include medication and psychotherapy. Major depression is diagnosed if at least five of the following symptoms have been present during the same two-week period:

- Depression which lasts most of the day, nearly every day.
- Diminished interest or pleasure in most activities every day.
- Significant change in weight or appetite.
- Daily insomnia or feeling the need to sleep all of the time.
- Psychomotor agitation or retardation.
- Fatigue or loss of energy.
- Feelings of worthlessness or excessive guilt.
- Diminished ability to think or concentrate.
- Recurrent thoughts of death or suicide.

## • Dysthymia

While this form of depression is milder, it is chronic, lasting for two years or more. Although most people with this disorder continue to function at work or school, they are often going through the motions and not taking any pleasure in life's activities. Dysthymia is treated with both antidepressants and psychotherapy. It is diagnosed if at least two of the following symptoms are present for a minimum of two years:

- Poor appetite or overeating.
- Insomnia or sleeping all the time.
- Low energy or fatigue.
- Low self-esteem.
- Poor concentration or an inability to make decisions.
- Feelings of hopelessness.

## • Adjustment Disorder with Depressed Mood

Generally, people suffering from this type of depression have a precipitating event that begins the depression, such as losing a job or ending an intimate relationship. Many people are able to recover from adjustment disorders on their own. The condition is diagnosed if most of the following are present:

- A reaction to an identifiable stressor that occurred within three months of the depression.
- Impairment in functioning at school, at work, or in social relationships.
- Symptoms in excess of a normal reaction to the stressor.
- The disturbance is not merely one instance of a pattern of overreaction to stress.
- The maladaptive reaction persists no longer than six months.
- The disturbance does not meet the criteria for any specific mental disorder.

## Diagnosing Depression: Rule Out Associated Conditions

In addition to using the criteria listed above to diagnose depression, a health care practitioner must rule out other conditions that may be linked to depressive states. These include:

### • Hypothyroidism

Hypothyroidism develops slowly in most individuals, taking many months or even years to become full-blown. It is characterized by lethargy and decreased sexual interest, among other things, in addition to an inability to regulate body temperature, dry skin, and constipation. Because some of these symptoms are common in patients with depression, too, it is necessary to conduct laboratory tests to rule out the possibility of hypothyroidism in a person who seems to be suffering from depression. The best way to do this is through laboratory tests that can analyze the different forms of the thyroid hormone and thyroid-stimulating hormone as well as antibodies in the blood.

### • Hypercalcemia

This condition, which is diagnosed by laboratory tests and characterized by raised serum calcium, may be caused by a malignancy that has spread to the bones. Hypercalcemia can also be a result of hyperparathyroidism, a condition in which one or more of the parathyroid glands produces an overabundance of their hormone, causing calcium concentrations in the blood to rise. Hypercalcemia may be confused with depression because both cause symptoms of indefinite fatigue and general list-lessness.

### • Pancreatic Cancer

The possibility of pancreatic cancer should be ruled out in diagnosing depression, particularly among elderly patients who report a new onset of depression, decreased appetite, and weight loss. They may also exhibit jaundice, an abnormal yellow appearance to the skin. Diagnosis of pancreatic cancer should be made only by an experienced physician.

### • Vitamin Deficiencies

A number of vitamin deficiencies, especially in B12 and folic acid, result in many of the same mood changes and behaviors associated with depression. It is important to rule these out, as vitamin deficiencies are readily treated with supplements, alleviating the patient's depressive symptoms.

### • Parkinson's Disease

Nearly half of all patients diagnosed with Parkinson's disease also suffer from depression. Symptoms of depression may occur early in the course of Parkinson's, even prior to the onset of classical motor symptoms.

## The First Step to Take in Treating Depression: Ensure a Healthy Diet and Incorporate an Exercise Regimen

Dietary intake may be severely compromised in depression, as individuals with depression are likely to experience significant changes in appetite. From anorexia to poor eating habits, depression sets the stage for a malnourished state. One study, published in 1994 in the *Journal of the American College of Nutrition*, reported that individuals diagnosed with moderate to severe depression had such poor dietary intake that they suffered from demonstrated deficiencies in a number of important nutrients.

Therefore, one of the first steps anyone diagnosed with depression can take toward health is to follow the guidelines we set forth earlier, in the complete *Brain Wellness Plan* nutrition guidelines. This plan includes a number of important supplements with proven benefits in treating depression, particularly the B vitamins.

In addition, we recommend that people diagnosed with depression work with a health care professional in adding a regular exercise routine, as exercise has been shown to raise serotonin levels in the brain. Patients should also consider the role sugar and hypoglycemia in contributing to depressive symptoms (see below).

## Nutritional Supplements You Can Begin Incorporating Now

### • Chromium and Vanadium: These Regulating Nutrients Help Restore Fluctuating Blood Sugar Levels

The brain is highly dependent on glucose as a major energy source. Fluctuations in blood sugar, therefore, may result in behavioral changes and aggravate depression. These fluctuations may be caused by either insulin resistance—a condition where the cells of your body are unable to accept the role of insulin to provide glucose—or metabolic disturbances.

For example, University of Philadelphia researchers have used PET scans to view the way that the brains of individuals with late-life depression metabolize glucose. These individuals showed widespread reductions in their ability to metabolize glucose in various areas of their brains.

Another study from the same institution examined the association between depression and alterations in glucose use. Through a five-hour glucose test, two groups of individuals—one diagnosed with depression, one not—were asked to fast and then take a sugar solution. Following that, the scientists took serial measurements of the blood sugar levels among all participants. The results showed that patients diagnosed with depression exhibited significantly higher glucose levels, greater cumulative glucose responses, and larger insulin responses compared to healthy individuals.

These and other studies indicate that many individuals with depression suffer from insulin resistance and disturbed glucose control. We recommend that people with depression avoid sugar and sugar products, and focus their dietary intake around a higher protein, lower carbohydrate regimen taken in frequent small meals.

In addition, we suggest incorporating supplements of chromium and vanadium to assist in regulating blood sugar levels.

**RECOMMENDED DOSES:**

| | |
|---|---|
| Chromium | 200 mcg twice daily, with meals (Take a fully reacted mineral chelate.) |
| Vanadium | 500 mcg daily, with a meal. (Look for the vanadyl sulfate form.) |

## • Fatty Acids: Cell Membrane Strengtheners Assist in Neurotransmitter Function

As we have seen earlier in this chapter, depression may be partly the result of increased consumption of the saturated fats found in meat and diary products, as well as our overreliance on the omega-6 polyunsaturated fatty acids in corn and safflower oil. This, coupled with a deficient intake of the essential omega-3 fatty acids, can significantly impair brain function and lead to depression.

We recommend that individuals diagnosed with depression boost their intake of omega-3 fatty acids to build strong brain cell membranes and improve their ability to synthesize, release, and bind with neurotransmitters such as serotonin. You can do this by adding supplements of MaxEPA™, DHA, and flaxseed oil.

*RECOMMENDED DAILY DOSES:*

| | |
|---|---|
| MaxEPA™ | 2 g |
| DHA | 300 mg |

(Look for the trademarked Neuromins™ from Martek Biosciences Corporation.)

| | |
|---|---|
| Flaxseed oil (organic, cold-pressed, keep refrigerated) | 1 tbsp |

All supplements are to taken with food.

## • One More Fatty Acid: Add Phosphatidylserine (PS) to Build up Cell Membranes

As we have seen throughout this book, our brain health depends on PS more than on any other single fatty acid. Besides maintaining and improving brain cell membranes, PS is essential for cells to efficiently metabolize glucose for energy and successfully release and bind with neurotransmitters. PS also serves as an added barrier against antioxidants pummeling our brain cell membranes. Patients diagnosed with clinical depression have shown marked improvement in symptoms as a result of taking PS daily.

Currently, PS is available from soy lecithin extract in 100 mg softgels.

**RECOMMENDED DOSE:** 300 mg daily (look for the trade-marked Leci-PS™ from Lucas Meyer).

## • Inositol: A Valuable Second Messenger

As we have seen, neurotransmitters cause a chain of chemical reactions in brain cells by binding to cell membranes and provoking a reaction that involves "second messenger" chemicals. These wily second messengers can cross the cell membrane and provoke reactions within the cells themselves.

One of the most valuable precursors to manufacturing these second messengers is inositol, which studies have shown is reduced in the cerebrospinal fluid of many depressed patients.

At the Ministry of Health Center at Ben Gurion University in Israel, researchers demonstrated that supplements of inositol successfully reduced depression among patients who were previously unresponsive to antidepressants. In addition, scientists at Israel's Abarbanel Mental Health Center have shown that depressed patients improved after taking 12 g of inositol daily, and relapsed after they discontinued the supplements.

Because ot its marked antidepressant effects and its safe, non-toxic nature, we recommend incorporating supplements of inositol to treat depression.

RECOMMENDED DOSE: 6–12 g daily, divided throughout the day. The lower dose range may be successful if using other natural agents in a total nutritional protocol, as outlined in this chapter.

## •Additional Nutritional Substances to Consider with Your Health Care Practitioner

## • SAM: Increase Serotonin and Norepinephrine Levels to Ease Symptoms of Depression

A number of studies in Great Britain, Italy, and the United States have shown that the natural substance SAM (s-adenosyl methionine) acts as an antidepressant. SAM supplements have been shown to increase concentrations of the two most important mood-altering neurotransmitters, serotonin and norepinephrine, and may prove to be a useful antidepressant particularly for those patients who cannot tolerate the side effects of standard antidepressants.

In using SAM as a therapeutic agent to treat depression, for example, researchers at the University of California at Los Angeles discovered that SAM acted as a rapid, effective antidepressant with very few side effects. In a paper published in the *American Journal of Psychiatry,* these scientists suggest that SAM's influence on phospholipid metabolism may be the principal explanation for its antidepressant effects, as SAM increases the fluidity of brain cell membranes and can affect the way in which brain cells receive and transmit neurotransmitters such as serotonin.

*RECOMMENDED DOSE:* Consult with your health care practitioner about sources, dosages, and ongoing studies.

## • Tryptophan: An Essential Ingredient for Your Body to Manufacture Serotonin

Scientific literature has repeatedly reported that depression is generally accompanied by a lower availability of tryptophan to the brain. Researchers have concluded that this amino acid is an essential precursor to your body's ability to manufacture serotonin.

Many years ago, tryptophan was taken off the market because of some contaminated material that caused serious illness among those individuals who consumed it. This problem was isolated to one manufacturer, and the contaminant was subsequently identified. Unfortunately, L-tryptophan is still not allowed for sale and may be obtained only by prescription, despite the fact that it is an essential amino acid and has been incorporated into infant formulas and hospital parenteral feedings.

In summary, then, the use of tryptophan in treating depression is still under investigation, and may even be harmful if tryptophan is combined with SSRIs. We urge patients considering tryptophan should do so only under the care of a skilled nutritionist or nutritionally oriented physician.

## • The Role of St. John's Wort as an Herbal Antidepressant

St. John's wort is a perennial that has received a great deal of attention over the past decade in treating viral conditions in immuno-compromised patients. Two of the plant's active ingredients, hypericin and xanthrones, have been shown to be monoamine oxidase (MAO) inhibitors.

MAO inhibitors are commonly used to treat depression. They function by literally reducing the levels of the monoamine ozidase enzyme, the enzyme responsible for breaking down neurotransmitters such as serotonin and norepinephrine. In effect, MAO inhibitors cause levels of these neurotransmitters to rise, because they are not so rapidly broken down and dispersed as by-products.

In studies examining the worth of St. John's wort as an antidepressant, investigators reporting in *The British Medical Journal* concluded that trials comparing this herb to a placebo showed that St. John's wort extracts are effective in treating mild to moderately severe depressive disorders. We suggest working with a nutrition-ist to explore the benefits of this herb in your own regime, beginning with smaller dosages and gradually increasing to assess any sensitivities.

RECOMMENDED DOSE: 300 mg daily as an initial dose. Look for a standarized St. John's wort extract. As with any herb, long-term usage must be assessed with your health care practitioner.

## Antidepressant Medications

As we mentioned earlier, about two-thirds of all individuals diagnosed with depression are likely to respond well to one of the antidepressant medications. People taking antidepressants generally feel the depressive symptoms gradually lift; they are still able to feel sadness or joy at appropriate times. In other words, antidepressants are not happy pills. At best, these medica-tions simply relieve depression and allow individuals to return to their normal activities and enjoy life again.

There are many classes of antidepressants. Two of them, the tricyclic antidepressants and the monoamine oxidase inhibitors, have been used successfully for decades. The most popular new class of antidepressants are the selective serotonin reuptake inhib-itors (SSRIs). Most recently, venlafaxine (Effexor) was added to the roster of available antidepressants.

We have listed the most commonly prescribed antidepressants below. Naturally, you should discuss proper administration, drug interactions, and the potential benefits and side effects of each with your health care practitioner.

The important thing to remember here is that, even if the first antidepressant you try does not relieve symptoms after several weeks, there is another that will most likely work.

- *Tricyclic Antidepressants*
  imipramine (Tofranil)

amitriptyline (Elavil)
nortriptyline (Aventyl and Pamelor)
desipramine (Norpramin)

- *Monoamine Oxidase Inhibitors*
tranylcypromine (Parnate)
phenelzine (Nardil)

- *Selective Serotonin Reuptake Inhibitors*
fluoxetine (Prozac)
sertraline (Zoloft)
paroxetine (Paxil)
fluvoxamine (Luvox)

- *Others*
bupropion (Wellbutrin)
traxodone (Desyrel)
venlafaxine (Effexor)

## Putting It All Together

Because Doreen was so intent on avoiding antidepressant medication, we suggested that she continue her therapy and work with a nutritionist to incorporate the nutrients described in *The Brain Wellness Plan* into her diet. In addition, we suggested that she join one of the intramural basketball teams, as she had always enjoyed the sport and we knew that the exercise would naturally raise her serotonin levels.

Doreen began increasing her consumption of the omega-3 fatty acids that first year, adding a 300 mg supplement of phosphatidylserine daily, as well as MaxEPA™, DHA, and flaxseed oil. Additionally, we asked Doreen to incorporate inositol and a small trial run of standardized St. John's wort.

Gradually, Doreen's depression has improved over the past two years to the point where she has only infrequent, mild episodes that no longer interfere with her ability to study or enjoy sports. She has resumed her full-time class schedule.

Now that you have an overview of depression and understand how this pervasive disease affects brain metabolism and function, you are no doubt eager to begin—or to help someone you know begin—to investigate the ways in which you can restore optimum levels of mood-altering neurotransmitters such as serotonin and norepinephrine in your brain.

Here is our summary guideline for treatment.

*Daily Nutritional Supplements*

| | |
|---|---|
| MaxEPA™ | 2 g |
| DHA | 300 mg (Look for trademarked Neuromins™ from Matek Biosciences Corporation.) |
| Flaxseed oil (organic, cold-pressed, keep refrigerated) | 1 tbsp |
| PS (phosphatidylserine) | 300 mg (Look for trademarked Leci-PS™ from Lucas Meyer.) |
| Inositol | 6 to 12 g daily, in divided doses. |
| St. John's wort | 300 mg as an initial dose. Consult with a nutritionist about increasing dosage. |

*In Case of Glucose Intolerance*

| | |
|---|---|
| Chromium | 200 mcg with meals (Look for a fully reacted chelate.) |
| Vanadium | 500 mcg with meals (Look for the vanadyl sulfate form.) |

*Additional Nutritional Substances to Consider with Your Health Care Practitioner*

SAM (s-adenosyl methionine)

Consult with your health care practitioner about sources and dosages.

*Medications*

See detailed list above.

# RESOURCES

## PROFESSIONAL ORGANIZATIONS

The following organizations offer additional information and support to patients and their families.

*Alzheimer's*
Alzheimer's Association
70 East Lake Street
Suite 600
Chicago, IL 60601
(312) 853-3060
(800) 621-0379

*Parkinson's*
National Parkinson's
Foundation
1501 Northwest Ninth Avenue
Bob Hope Road
Miami, FL 33136
(305) 547-6666
(800) 327-4545

Parkinson's Disease
Foundation
Columbia-Presbyterian
Medical Center
650 West 168th Street
New York, NY 10032
(800) 457-6676

*Multiple Sclerosis*
National Multiple Sclerosis
Society
733 Third Avenue
New York, NY 10017
(212) 986-3240
(800) 624-8232

*Amyotrophic Lateral Sclerosis*
The ALS Association
21021 Ventura Boulevard
Suite 321
Woodland Hills, CA 91364
(818) 340-7500
(800) 782-4747

*Attention Deficit Hyperactivity Disorder*
CHADD
1859 North Pine Island Road
Suite 185
Plantation, FL 33322
(954) 587-3700

*Chronic Fatigue Syndrome*
CFIDS of America
P.O. Box 220398
Charlotte, NC 28222
(800) 442-3437

*Depression*
National Foundation for
  Depressive Illnesses
P.O. Box 2257
New York, NY 10116
(800) 248-4344

## NUTRITIONAL ASSOCIATIONS

The following is a list of professional organizations that will serve as useful resources of information on herbs, nutrition, and preventive medical care.

American Botanical Council
P.O. Box 201660
Austin, TX 78720-1660
(512) 331-8868;
fax (512) 331-1924

American College of
  Alternative Medicine
(800) 532-3688

American Holistic Medical
  Association
4101 Lake Boone Trail, Suite
  201
Raleigh, NC 27607
(919) 787-5146

American Preventive Medical
  Association
P.O. Box 2111
Tacoma, WA 98401
(206) 926-0551;
fax (206) 922-7583

Citizens for Health
P.O. Box 2260
Boulder, CO 80306-1195
(303) 417-0772;
fax (303) 417-9378

Council for Responsible
  Nutrition (CRN)
1300 Nineteenth Street NW,
  Suite 310
Washington, DC 20036-1609
(202) 872-1488

Herb Research Foundation
1007 Pearl Street, Suite 200
Boulder, CO 80302-5124
(303) 449-2265;
fax (303) 449-7849

## NUTRITIONAL SUPPLEMENT RESOURCES

The following is a partial listing of nutritional supplement companies that sell many of the items recommended in the book.

### Retail Health Food Store Brands

Solgar Vitamin & Herb
  Company, Inc.
World Headquarters
500 Willow Tree Road
Leonia, NJ 07605
(201) 944-2311;
fax (201) 944-7351
http://www.solgar.com

Carlson Laboratories, Inc.
15 W. College Drive
Arlington Heights, IL 60004
(847) 255-1600
fax (847) 255-1605

Nature's Plus, Inc.
548 Broad Hollow Road
Melville, NY 11747
(516) 293-0030;
fax (516) 293-0349

*Medically Oriented Brands—Mail Order/Direct Sales*

United Nutraceuticals, Inc.
*Total Brain Wellness*™
*Total Brain Nutrition*™
23 Vreeland Road, Suite 104
Florham Park, NJ 07932
(800) 434-0447;
fax (201) 822-0335

Metagenics, Inc.
971 Calle Negocio
San Clemente, CA 92673-6202
(714) 366-0818;
fax (714) 366-2859

Ultimate Health, Inc.
215 North Route 303
Congers, NY 10920
(800) 292-6002;
fax (914) 268-2988

# FOOD SOURCES FOR THE BRAIN WELLNESS NUTRIENTS RECOMMENDED THROUGHOUT THE BOOK

**None of the foods listed can be eaten in sufficient amounts to elicit a nutritional therapeutic effect, and therefore, we do recommend supplements.** However, these foods do provide the basis for a healthy diet and optimum brain wellness.

| Nutrient | Food Sources |
| --- | --- |
| Phosphatidylserine (PS) | Lecithin |
| Docosahexaneoic Acid (DHA) | Fatty fish, fish oil |
| Genistein | Soy foods, soy protein |
| NAC (n-acetyl-cysteine) | Protein foods, such as fish and poultry |
| ALC (acetyl-L-carnitine) | Protein foods, such as fish |
| Glutamine | Protein foods, such as fish |
| Threonine | Protein foods, such as fish and poultry |
| Lipoic Acid | Liver, yeast |
| Polyphenols, proanthocyanidins | Red wine; green tea; fruit, grapes; grape seed and pine bark extracts; and herbs such as bilberry, ginkgo, and milk thistle. |

Vitamin E

| | |
|---|---|
| Tocopherols | Polyunsaturated vegetable oils, seeds, nuts |
| Tocotrienols | Barley and rice oils |
| Coenzyme Q10 | Every plant and animal cell |
| Vitamin C | Citrus fruits, broccoli, peppers, and other dark-colored vegetables and fruits |

B vitamins

| | |
|---|---|
| Thiamine | Brown rice, soybeans, seeds, yeast |
| Riboflavin | Yeast, organ meats, almonds, wheat germ |
| Niacin | Eggs, organ meats, fish, brown rice, seeds |
| B6 | Seeds, whole grains, beans, bananas, nuts |
| Biotin | Cheese, soybeans, organ meats, brown rice |
| Pantothenic acid | Fish, poultry, milk, nuts, soybeans, brown rice |
| Folic acid | Green leafy vegetables, beans, wheat germ, nuts |
| B12 | Organ meats, milk, fish, cheese, meat |
| Choline | Grains, beans, cauliflower, whole grains, lettuce |
| Inositol | Whole grains, citrus fruits, nuts, seeds, beans |

Minerals

| | |
|---|---|
| Calcium | Dairy products, tofu, kale, green leafy vegetables, seaweed |
| Magnesium | Tofu, beans, seeds, nuts, whole grains, green leafy vegetables |

| | |
|---|---|
| Zinc | Shellfish, fish, meats, whole grains, beans, seeds |
| Manganese | Nuts, whole grains, dried fruits, green leafy vegetables |
| Selenium | Wheat germ, nuts, whole grains, Swiss chard, garlic |
| Vanadium | Parsley, mushrooms, shellfish, soybeans, corn |
| Carotenoids: alpha and beta | Carrots, tomatoes, squash, kale |
| Carotene, lutein, lycopene | Collards, broccoli, yams, other dark-colored fruits and vegetables |

# REFERENCES

## Part I

### • Chapter One: Brain-Immune Connection Basics

Bindoni M., et al. Interleukin-2 modifies the bioelectrical activity of some neurosecretory nuclei in the rat hypothalamus. Brain Res 1988; 462: 10–14.

Black P. Psychoneuroimmunology. Brain and immunity. Scientific American 1995 Nov–Dec: 16–25.

Blum F. and Kupfer D., eds. Psychopharmacology, the Fourth Generation of Progress. Raven Press, 1995.

Carpenter M., ed. Core Text of Neuroanatomy, 4th ed. Williams and Wilkins, 1991.

Fabris N., Markovic B.M., Spector N.H., Jankovic B.D., eds. Neuroimmunomodulations: the state of the art. Ann NY Acad Sci 1994; Vol. 741.

Ganong W.F., Dallman M.F., Roberts J.L., eds. The hypothalamic pituitary adrenal revisited. Ann NY Acad Sci 1987; Vol. 512.

Jankovic B.D., Markovic B.M., Spector N.H., eds. Neuroimmune interactions. Ann NY Acad Sci 1987; Vol. 496.

Netter F. Ciba Collection of Medical Illustrations. Nervous System Anatomy and Physiology, Vol. 1. Ciba-Geigy, 1991.

Scriver C.R., Beaudet A.L., Sly W.S., Valle D.S., eds. Metabolic and Molecular Bases of Inherited Disease, 7th ed. McGraw-Hill Inc., 1995.

Shatz, C. The developing brain. Sci American 1992 Sept; 267(3): 60–7.

Snyder S. Nitric oxide: first in a new class of neurotransmitter. Science 1992 Jul; Vol. 253.

Streight W.J. and Kincaid-Colton C.A. The brain's immune system. Sci American 1995 Nov; 273 (5): 54–61.

• *Chapter Two: Communication Breakdown*

Barinaga M. Cell suicide: by ICE, not FIRE. Science 1994 Feb. 11; 263: 754–6.

Beal M.F. Aging, energy and oxidative stress in neurodegenerative diseases. Ann Neurol 1995 Sept; 38(3): 357–68.

Chan T.H. and Fishman R.A. Free fatty acids, oxygen free radicals and membrane alterations and brain ischemia and injury. In Cerebrovascular Disease, Plum F. and Pulsinell W., eds. Raven Press, 1985: 161–71.

Heyes M.P. Relationship between interferon gamma, indoleamine, #2-3 dioxygenase and tryptophans. FASEB J 1991; 5: 3003–4.

Murphy T., et al. Arachidonic acid metabolism in glutamate neurotoxicity in arachidonic metabolism in the nervous system. Ann NY Acad Sci 1989; 559.

Olanow C.W. A radical hypothesis for neurodegeneration. Trends in Neuroscience 1993; 16: 439–44.

Oldstone M.B. Molecular mimicry and autoimmune disease. Zell 1987 Sept; 50(6): 819–20.

Opp M.R., et al. Cytokine involvement in the regulation of sleep. Proc Soc Exp Biol Med 1992; 201: 16–27.

Palmer A.M., Burns M. Selective increase in lipid peroxidation in the inferior temporal cortex in Alzheimer's disease. Brain Res 1994; 645: 338–47.

Rothstein J., et al. Chronic inhibition of the superoxide dismutase produces apoptotic death of spinal neurons. Proc Nat Acad of Sci 1994 May; 91: 4155–9.

Rubbo H., et al. Nitric oxide regulation of superoxide and peroxynitrate dependent lipid peroxidation. J of Biol Chem 1994; 269(42): 26066–75.

Sapolsky R.M., et al. Inhibition of glucocorticoid secretion by the hippocampal formation in the primate. J of Neuroscience 1991; 11: 3695–704.

Steinman L. Autoimmune disease. Sci American 1993 Sept; 107–14.

Vandenabelle P., et al. Is amyloidogenesis during Alzheimer's disease due to IL-1/Il-6 mediated acute phase response in the brain? Immunol Today 1991; 12: 217–9.

## • Chapter Three: Food for Thought

Ahnert-Hilger G. and Bigalke H. Molecular aspects of tetanus and botulinum neurotoxin poisoning. Progress in Neurobiology 1995; 46: 83–96.

Bland J. New perspectives in nutritional therapies. Health Com. Inc., 1996.

Dawks D. Disorders of copper transport. In Metabolic and Molecular Bases of Inherited Diseases, 7th ed., Vol 2. Scriver C., Beaudet A., Sly W. and Valle D., eds. McGraw-Hill Inc., 1995.

Eastwood S.L. and Harrison P.J. Decreased synaptophysin in the medial temporal lobe in schizophrenia demonstrated using immunoautoradiography. Letters to Neuroscience 1995; 69: 339–343.

Frederickson C.J. Neurobiology of zinc and zinc-containing neurons. Rev Neurobiol 1989; 31: 146–238.

Gibson R.S., et al. A growth-limiting, mild zinc deficiency syndrome in some South Ontario boys with low height percentiles. Am J of Clin Nutrition 1991; 49: 1266–73.

Huan Y., et al. Further study on the magnesium-mediated change in physical state of phospholipid modulates mitochondrial ATP ASE activity. Magnesium Res 1993; 6: 321–7.

Krieger D., Bronstein M., Martin J., eds. Brain Peptides. John Wiley and Sons Inc., 1983.

Lindenbaum J., et al. Neuropsychiatric disorders caused by cobalamin deficiency in the absence of anemia or macrocytosis. N Engl J Med 1988 Jun 30; 318(26): 1720–8.

Lockwood A.H. Hepatic encephalopathy and other neurological diseases associated with gastrointestinal disease. In Neurology and General Medicine, Aminoff M. ed. Churchill Livingston Publishing, 1989.

Magistretti P.J., Pellerin L., Martin J.L. Brain energy metabolism: an integrative cellular perspective. In Psychopharmacology: The Fourth Generation of Progress. Bloom F. and Kupfer D., eds. Raven Press, 1995.

Ramadan N. and Welch K. Migraine and cluster headaches. In Current Therapy in Neurological Diseases, 4th ed., Johnson R. and Griffin J., eds. Mosby Yearbook, 1990.

Rowland L. Nutritional deficiency in gastrointestinal disease. In Merrits Textbook of Neurology, 8th ed., Rowland L. ed. Lea & Bebiger Publishing, 1989.

Shaw W., et al. Increased urinary excretion of analogs of krebs scyle metabolites and arabinose in two brothers with autistic features. Clin Chem 1995; 1094–104.

• Chapter Four: The Brain Wellness Plan

Agostoni C., et al. Neurodevelopmental quotients of healthy term infants at 4 months and feeding practice: the role of long-chain polyunsaturated fatty acids. Ped Res 1994 Aug; 38: 262–6.

Asahi M., Fujii J., Suzuki K., Seo H.G., et al. Inactivation of glutathione peroxidase by nitric oxide. Implication for cytotoxicity. J Biol Chem 1995 Sept 8; 270(36): 21035-9.

Baldessarini R.J. The neuropharmacology of S-adenosyl methionine. Am J of Med 1987; 83: 95–103.

Barbiroli B., Medori R., Tritschler H.J., et al. Lipoic (thioctic) acid increases brain energy availability and skeletal muscle performance as shown by in vivo 31P-MRS in a patient with mitochondrial cytopathy. J Neurol 1995 Jul; 242(7): 472–7.

Barbour B. Arachidonic acid induces a prolonged inhibition of glutamate uptake into glial cells. Nature 1989; 342: 918–20.

Bottigleri T. Cerebrospinal fluid S-adenosyl methionine in depression and dementia: effects of treatment with parenteral and oral S-adenosyl methionine. J of Neurol, Neurosurg and Psych 1990; 53: 1056–98.

Boutard V., Fouqueray B., Philippe C., et al. Fish oil supplementation and essential fatty acid deficiency reduce nitric oxide synthesis by rat macrophages. Kidney Int 1994 Nov; 46(5): 1280–6.

Duval D.L., Sieg D.J., Billings R.E. Regulation of hepatic nitric oxide synthase by reactive oxygen intermediates and glutathione. Arch Biochim Biophys 1995 Feb 1; 316(2): 699–706.

Fridel H.A., et al. S-adenosyl methionine. A review of its pharmacological properties and therapeutic potential in liver dysfunction and affective disorders in relation to its physiological role in cell metabolism. Drugs 1989; 38: 389–416.

Gaiti, A. The Aging Brain. Arachadonic Acid Metabolism in the Nervous System. Barkai A. and Bazan N.G., eds. Ann NY Acad Sci, Vol. 559: 1989.

Hall E. Free radicals and CNS injury. Crit Care Clinics 1989 Oct; 5(4): 793–805.

Han D., Tritschler H.J., Packer L. Alpha-lipoic acid increases intracellular glutathione in a human T-lymphocyte Jurkat cell line. Biochim Biophys Res Commun 1995 Feb 6; 207(1): 258–64.

Hellerstein M.K., Wu K., McGrath M., et al. Effects of dietary n-3 fatty acid supplementation in men with weight loss associated with the acquired immune deficiency syndrome: relation to indices of cytokine production. J Acquir Immune Defic Syndr Hum Retrovirol 1996 Mar 1; 11(3): 258–70.

Hogg N., Singh R.J., Kalyanaraman B. The role of glutathione in the transport and catabolism of nitric oxide. FEBS Lett 1996 Mar 18; 382(3): 223–8.

Justaffson L.E. Mechanisms involved in the action of prostaglandins as modulators of neurotransmission. Ann NY Acad Sci 1989; 559: 178–91.

Kiens B., Rasmussen L.B., Pedersen B.K., Richter E.A. Significance of fatty acid composition in plasma and in food for cellular immune function in elderly men. Ugeskr Laeger 1994 Oct 24; 156(43): 6388–91.

Kuo P.C. and Abe K.Y. Nitric oxide-associated regulation of hepatocyte glutathione synthesis is a guanylyl cyclase-independent event. Surgery 1996 Aug; 120(2): 309–14.

Lizasoain I., Moro M.A., Knowles R.G., et al. Nitric oxide and peroxynitrite exert distinct effects on mitochondrial respiration which are differentially blocked by glutathione or glucose. Biochem J 1996 Mar 15; 314(Pt 3): 877–80.

Majewska M., et al. Neuronal action of DHEA: possible role in brain development, aging and memory. Ann NY Acad Sci 1994; 774: 11–12.

Mayer M. and Noble M. N-acetyl-L-cysteine is a pluripotent protector against cell death and enhancer of trophic factor-mediated cell survival in vitro. Proc Natl Acad Sci 1994 Aug 2; 91(16): 7496–500.

Miller B., et al. Potentiation of NMDA receptor currents by arachidonic acid. Nature 1992; 355: 722–5.

Moore S.A., et al. Role of the blood-brain barrier in the formation of long chain omega-3 and omega-6 fatty acids from essential fatty acid precursors. J of Neurochem 1990; 55: 391–402.

Muller U. and Krieglstein J. Prolonged pretreatment with alpha-lipoic acid protects cultured neurons against hypoxic-glutamate-, or iron-induced injury. J Cereb Blood Flow Metab 1995 Jul; 15(4): 624–30.

Ordway R.W., et al. Direct regulation of ion channels by fatty acids. Trends in Neuroscience 1001; 14: 96–100.

Orentreich N., et al. Long-term measurement of plasma DHEA sulfate in normal men. J of Clin Endocrin and Metabolism 1992; 75: 1002–5.

Packer L., Witt E.H., Tritschler H.J. Alpha-lipoic acid as a biological antioxidant. Free Rad Biol Med 1995 Aug; 19(2): 227–50.

Pani A., Marongiu M.E., La Colla P. Modulatory effect of N-acetyl-L-cysteine on the HIV-1 multiplication in chronically and acutely infected cell lines. Antiviral Res 1993 Sept; 22(1): 31–43.

Petit J.F., Nicaise M., Lepoivre M., et al. Protection by glutathione against the antiproliferative effects of nitric oxide. Biochem Pharmacol 1996 Jul 26; 52(2): 205–12.

Pettegrew J.W., et al. Clinical and neurochemical effects of acetyl-L-carnitine in Alzheimer's disease. Neurobiol of Aging 1995 Jan-Feb; 16(1–4).

Rasmussen L.B., Kiens B., Pedersen B.K., Richter E.A. Effect of diet and plasma fatty acid composition on immune status in elderly men. Am J Clin Nutr 1994 Mar; 59(3): 572–9.

Regelson W. Dehydroepiandrostone (DHEA), the multi-functional steroid: effects on the central nervous system, cell proliferation, metabolic and vascular clinical and other effects. Ann NY Acad Sci 1994; 564: 564–75.

Scarlett J.L., Packer M.A., Porteous C.M., Murphy M.P. Alterations to glutathione and nicotinamide nucleotides during the mitochondrial permeability transition induced by peroxynitrite. Biochem Pharmacol 1996 Oct 11; 52(7): 1047–55.

Scott B.C., Aruoma O.I., Evans P.J., et al. Lipoic and dihydrolipoic acids as antioxidants. A critical evaluation. Free Radic Res 1994 Feb; 20(2): 119–33.

Shibanuma M., Kuroki T., Nose K. Inhibition by N-acetyl-L-cysteine of interleukin-6 mRNA induction and activation of NF kappa B by tumor necrosis factor alpha in a mouse fibroblastic cell line, Balb/3T3. FEBS Lett 1994 Oct 10; 353(1): 62–6.

Van der Vliet A., Smith D., O'Neill C.A., et al. Interactions of peroxynitrite with human plasma and its constituents: oxidative damage and antioxidant depletion. Biochem J 1994 Oct 1; 303 (Pt. 1): 295–301.

Vatassery G.T. Oxidation of vitamin E, vitamin C, and thiols in rat brain synaptosomes by peroxynitrite. Biochem Pharmacol 1996 Aug 23; 52(4): 579–86.

Walker M.W., Kinter M.T., Roberts R.J., Spitz D.R. Nitric oxide—induced cytotoxicity: involvement of cellular resistance to oxidative stress and the role of glutathione in protection. Ped Res 1995 Jan; 37(1): 41–9.

Weber P.C. Membrane phospholipid modification by dietary N-3 fatty acids: effects on eicosanoid formation and cell function in biological membranes. In Aberrations in Membrane Structure and Function, Liss A., ed., 1988: 263–74.

White A.C., Maloney E.K., Boustani M.R., et al. Nitric oxide increases cellular glutathione levels in rat lung fibroblasts. Am J Respir Cell Mol Biol 1995 Oct; 13(4): 442–8.

Whiteman M., Tritschler H., Halliwell B. Protection against peroxynitrite-dependent tyrosine nitration and alpha 1-antiproteinase inactivation by oxidized and reduced lipoic acid. FEBS Lett 1996 Jan 22; 379(1): 74–6.

# Part II

• Chapter Five: Alzheimer's Disease

Adams J.D., et al. Alzheimer's and Parkinson's disease brain levels of glutathione, glutathione disulfide, and vitamin E. Mol and Chem Neuropathol 1991; 14: 213–23.

Aisen P.S. and Davis K.L. Inflammatory mechanisms in Alzheimer's disease: implications for therapy. Am J Psychiatry 1994 Aug; 151(8): 1105–13.

Amaducci L. Phosphatidylserine in the treatment of Alzheimer's disease: results of a multicenter study. Psychopharmacol Bull 1988; 24(1): 130–4.

Amaducci L., Crook T.H., Lippi A., et al. Use of phosphatidylserine in Alzheimer's disease. Ann NY Acad Sci 1991; 640: 245–9.

Aureli T., Miccheli A., Ricciolini R., et al. Aging brain: effect of acetyl-L-carnitine treatment on rat brain energy and phospholipid metabolism. Brain Res 1990; 526: 108–12.

Bissette G., Seidler F.J., Nemeroff C.B., Slotkin T. High affinity choline transporter status in Alzheimer's disease tissue from rapid autopsy. Ann NY Acad Sci 1996 Jan 17; 777: 197–204.

Breitner J.C., Gau B.A., Welsh K.A., Plassman B.L., et al. Inverse association of anti-inflammatory treatments and Alzheimer's disease: initial results of a co-twin control study. Neurology 1994 Feb; 44(2): 227–32.

Brenner D.E., et al. Postmenopausal estrogen replacement therapy and the risk of Alzheimer's disease: population-based case-controlled study. Am J of Epidemiology 1994; 140; 262–7.

Bruno G., Scaccianoce S., Bonamini M., et al. Acetyl-L-carnitine in Alzheimer's disease: a short-term study on CSF neurotransmitters and neuropeptides. Alzheimer Dis Assoc Disord 1995 Fall; 9(3): 128–31.

Caamano J., Gomez J.J., Franco A., Cacabelos R. Effects of CDP-choline on cognition and cerebral hemodynamics in patients with Alzheimer's disease. Methods Find Exp Clin Pharmacol 1994 Apr; 16(3): 211–18.

Cacabelos R., Alvarez X.A., Franco-Maside A., Fernandez-Novoa L., Caamano J. Effect of CDP-choline on cognition and immune function in Alzheimer's disease and multi-infarct dementia. Ann NY Acad Sci 1993 Sept. 24; 695: 321–3.

Cacabelos R., Caamano J., Gomez M.J., Fernandez-Novoa L., et al. Therapeutic effects of CDP-choline in Alzheimer's disease. Cognition, brain mapping, cerebrovascular hemodynamics, and immune factors. Ann NY Acad Sci 1996 Jan 17; 777: 399–403.

Carta A., Calvani M., Bravi D., Bhuachalla S.N. Acetyl-L-carnitine and Alzheimer's disease: pharmacological considerations beyond the cholinergic sphere. Ann NY Acad Sci 1993 Sept. 24; 695: 324–6.

Castano E.M., Prelli F., Wisniewski T., Golabek A., et al. Fibrillogenesis in Alzheimer's disease of amyloid beta peptides and apolipoprotein E. Biochem J 1995 Mar 1; 306 (Pt. 2): 599–604.

Castorina M. and Ferraris L. Acetyl-L-carnitine affects aged brain receptorial system in rodents. Life Sci 1994; 54(17): 1205–14.

Cenacchi T., Bertoldin T., Farina C., et al. Cognitive decline in the elderly: a double-blind, placebo-controlled multicenter study on efficacy of phosphatidylserine administration. Aging 1993; 5: 123–33.

Cheney D.L., exec. ed. Pathology of Alzheimer's disease in: Neuroscience Facts 1991 Mar; 2(5): 1.

Crook T., Petrie W., Wells C., Casadei M.D. Effects of phosphatidylserine in Alzheimer's disease. Pharmacology Bull 1992; 28(1): 61–5.

Crook T.H., Tinklenberg J., et al. Effects of phosphatidylserine in age-associated memory impairment. Neurology 1991; 41: 644–9.

Davenport A. and Goodall R. Aluminum and dementia. Lancet 1992 May 16; 39: 1236.

Davis S., Markowska A.L., Wenk G.L., Barnes C.A. Acetyl-L-carnitine: behavioral, electrophysiological, and neurochemical effects. Neurobiol Aging 1993 Jan-Feb; 14(1): 107–15.

Dedman D., et al. Iron and aluminum in relation to brain ferritin in normal individuals and Alzheimer's disease and chronic renal dialysis patients. Biochem Journal 1992; 509–14.

De Feudis F.V. Ginkgo biloba extract (EGb 761): pharmacological activities and clinical applications. Elsevier, 1991.

Dumont E., D'Arbigny P., Nouvelot A. Protection of polyunsaturated fatty acids against iron-dependent lipid peroxidation by a ginkgo biloba extract (EGb 761). Methods Find Exp Clin Pharmacol 1995 Mar; 17(2): 83–8.

Eisinger J., et al. Erythrocyte transketolase in Alzheimer's disease: the thiamine hypothesis. J of the Advancement of Med 1994 Summer; 7(2): 69–75.

Engel R.R., Satzger W., Gunther W., et al. Double-blind crossover study of phosphatidylserine vs. placebo in patients with early dementia of the Alzheimer type. Eur Neuropsychopharmacol 1992 Jun; 2(2): 149–55.

Ershler W.B. Interleukin-6: a cytokine for gerontologists. JAGS 1993 Feb; 41(2): 176–81.

Farooqui A.A., Wells K., Horrorocks L.A. Breakdown of membrane phospholipids in Alzheimer's disease. Mol Chem Neuropathol 1995 Jun-Aug; 25(2–3): 155–73.

Fillit H. Estrogens in the pathogenesis and treatment of Alzheimer's disease in postmenopausal women. Ann NY Acad Sci 1994 Nov 14; 743: 223–8.

Forbes, et al. Aluminum and Alzheimer's disease. Can Med Assoc Journal 1992; 146(9): 1534.

Forloni G., Angeretti N., Smiroldo S. Neuroprotective activity of acetyl-L-carnitine: studies in vitro. J Neurosci Res 1994 Jan; 37(1): 92–6.

Franco-Maside A., Caamano J., Gomez M.J., Cacabelos R. Brain mapping activity and mental performance after chronic treatment with CDP-choline in Alzheimer's disease. Methods Find Exp Clin Pharmacol 1994 Oct; 16(8): 597–607.

Frolich L. and Riederer P. Free radical mechanisms in dementia of the Alzheimer's type and the potential for antioxidative treatment. Drug Res 1995; 45(1): 3A: 443–6.

Funfgeld E.W., Baggen M., Nedwidek P., et al. Double-blind study with phosphatidylserine (PS) in parkinsonian patients with senile dementia of Alzheimer's type (SDAT). Prog Clin Biol Res 1989; 317: 1235–46.

Gandy S.E., Bhasin R., Ramabhadran V., et al.: Alzheimer B/A4-amyloid precursor protein: evidence for putative amyloidogenic fragment. J Neurochem 1992; 58: 383–6.

Glick J. Dementias: the role of magnesium deficiency and hypothesis concerning the pathogenesis of Alzheimer's disease. Med Hypothesis 1990; 31: 211–25.

Gold M., et al. Plasma and red blood cell thiamine deficiency in patients with dementia of the Alzheimer's type. Arch Neurol 1995 Nov; 52: 1081–5.

Good P.F., Perl D.P., Bierer L.M., Schmeidler J. Selective accumulation of aluminum and iron in the neurofibrillary tangles of Alzheimer's disease: a laser microphobe (LAMMA) study. Ann of Neurol 1992 Mar; 31(3): 286–92.

Hardy J.A. and Higgins G.A. Alzheimer's disease: the amyloid cascade hypothesis. Science 1992 Apr 10; 256: 184–5.

Heiss W.D., Kessler J., Mielke R., et al. Long-term effects of phosphatidylserine, pyritinol, and cognitive training in Alzheimer's disease. A neuropsychological, EEG, and PET investigation. Dementia 1994 Mar-Apr; 5(2): 88–98.

Henderson V.W., Paganinin-Hill A., Emanuel C.K., Dun M.E., Buckwalter J.G. Estrogen replacement therapy in older women. Arch Neurol 1994 Sept; 51(9): 896–900.

Ikeda T., et al. Vitamin B12 levels in serum and cerebrospinal fluid of people with Alzheimer's disease. ACTA Psychiatr Scand 1990; 82: 327–9.

Imagawa M. Iron, B6 and coenzyme Q10 in Alzheimer's. The Nutrition Report 1994 Oct; 12(10): 75.

Imagawa M. Therapy with a combination of iron, vitamin B6 and coenzyme Q10 in the long term for sporadic Alzheimer's disease. Neurobiol 1994; A15: S101.

Imagawa M., et al. Coenzyme Q10, iron and vitamin B6 in genetically-confirmed Alzheimer's disease; Lancet 1992 Sept 12; 40: 671.

Jeandel C., et al. Lipid peroxidation and free radical scavengers in Alzheimer's disease. Gerontology 1989; 35: 275–82.

Johnson R. Estrogen/Alzheimer's link found. Medical Tribune 1993 Dec 9; 34(23): 1–8.

Kanowski S., et al. Proof of efficacy of the ginkgo biloba special extract EGb 761 in outpatients suffering from mild to moderate primary degenerative dementia of the Alzheimer type or multi-infarct dementia. Pharmacopsychiat 1996; 29: 47–56.

Klegeris A., Walker D.G., McGeer P.L. Activation of macrophages by Alzheimer beta amyloid peptide. Biochem Biophys Res Commun 1994 Mar 15; 199(2): 984–91.

Kose K. and Dogan P. Lipoperoxidation induced by hydrogen peroxide in human erythrocyte membrane. J Int Med Res 1995 Jan-Feb; 23(1): 1–8.

Kraus A.S. and Forbes W. Aluminum, fluoride and prevention of Alzheimer's disease. Can Journal of Public Health 1992 Mar-Apr; 83:(2): 97–100.

Kunkel H. EEG profile of three different extractions of ginkgo biloba. Neuropsychobiol 1993; 27(1): 40–5.

Levitt A.J., et al. Folate, vitamin B12 and cognitive impairment in patients with Alzheimer's disease. Acta Psychiatr Scand 1992; 86: 301–5.

Maitra I., Marcocci L., Droy-Lefaix M.T., Packer L. Peroxyl radical scavenging activity of ginkgo biloba extract EGb 761. Biochem Pharmacol 1995 May 26; 49(11): 1649–55.

Marcocci L., Maguire J.J., Droy-Lefaix M.T., Packer L. The nitric oxide–scavenging properties of ginkgo biloba extract EGb 761. Biochem Biophys Res Commun 1994 Jun 15; 201(2): 748–55.

Mason R.P., Trumbore M.W., Pettegrew J.W. Molecular membrane interactions of a phospholipid metabolite. Ann NY Acad Sci 1996 Jan 17; 777: 368–73.

Mastrogiacomo F., et al. Brain thiamine, its phosphate esters, and its metabolizing enzymes in Alzheimer's disease. Ann Neurol 1996; 39: 585–91.

McCaddon A. and Kelly C. Familial Alzheimer's disease and vitamin B12 deficiency. Age and Aging 1994 Jul; 23: 334–7.

McCaddon A. and Kelly C. Vitamin B12 and Alzheimer's disease. The Nutrition Report 1994 Oct; 12(10): 75.

McGeer P.L., McGeer E.G, Rogers J., Sibley J., Anti-inflammatory drugs and Alzheimer's disease. Lancet 1990; 335: 1037.

McGeer P.L. and Rogers J. Anti-inflammatory agents as a therapeutic approach to Alzheimer's disease. Neurology 1992; 42: 447–8.

Nolan K.A., et al. A trial of thiamine in Alzheimer's disease. Arch Neurol 1991 Jan; 48: 81–3.

Oyama Y., Hayashi A., Ueha T. Ca(2+)-induced increase in oxidative metabolism of dissociated mammalian brain neurons: effect of extract of ginkgo biloba leaves. Jpn J Pharmacol 1993 Apr; 61(4): 367–70.

Paganinin-Hill A; Henderson V.W. Estrogen deficiency and risk of Alzheimer's disease in women. Am J Epidemiol 1994 Aug 1; 140(3): 256–61.

Palmer A.M. and Burns M.A. Selective increase in lipid peroxidation in the inferior temporal cortex in Alzheimer's disease. Brain Res 1994 Feb; 645: 338–42.

Palmert M.R., Usiak B.S., Mayeux R., et al. Soluble derivatives of the B amyloid protein precursor in cerebrospinal fluid. Neurology 1990 Jul; 40: 1028–34.

Parnetti L., Gaiti A., Mecocci P., Senin U. Pharmacokinetics of IV and oral acetyl-L-carnitine in a multiple dose regimen in patients with senile dementia of Alzheimer type. Eur J Clin Pharmacol 1992; 42: 89–93.

Pettegrew J.W., Klunk W.E., Kanal E., et al. Changes in brain membrane phospholipid and high-energy phosphate metabolism precede dementia. Neurobiol Aging 1995 Nov-Dec; 16(6): 973–5.

Pettegrew J.W., Klunk W.E., Panchalingam K., Kanfer J.N., McClure R.J. Clinical and neurochemical effects of acetyl-L-carnitine in Alzheimer's disease. Neurobiol Aging 1995 Jan-Feb; 16(1): 1–4.

Pincemail J., Dupuis M., Nasr C., Hans P., et al. Superoxide anion scavenging effect and superoxide dismutase activity of ginkgo biloba extract. Experientia 1989 Aug 15; 45(8): 708–12.

Ren Z., Ding W., Su Z., Gu X., et al. Mechanisms of brain injury with deep hypothermic circulatory arrest and protective effects of coenzyme Q10. J Thorac Cardiovasc Surg 1994 Jul; 108(1): 126–33.

Rich J.B., Rasmusson D.X., Folstein M.F., Carson K.A. et al. Nonsteroidal anti-inflammatory drugs in Alzheimer's disease. Neurology 1995 Jan; 45(1): 51–5.

Robb-Nicholson C. and Merz B., eds. Estrogen and Alzheimer's Disease. Women's Health Watch 1996 Nov; Vol. IV (3): p. 1–3.

Rogers J. Inflammation as a pathogenic mechanism in Alzheimer's disease. Arzneimittel-Forschung/Drug Res 1995; 45(I), 3a, 439–42.

Rogers J., Kirby L.C., Hempelman S.R., et al. Clinical trial of indomethacin in Alzheimer's disease. Neurology 1993 Aug; 43: 1609–10.

Rogers S.L., Friedhoff L.T. and the Donepezil Study Group. Dementia 1996; 7: 293–303.

Sano M., Bell K., Cote L., et al. Double-blind parallel design pilot study of acetyl levocarnitine in patients with Alzheimer's disease. Arch Neurol 1992 Nov; 49: 1137–41.

Sano M. et al. A controlled trial of selegiline, alpha-tocopherol or both as treatment for Alzheimer's Disease. N Engl J Med 1997 Apr: 1216–1222.

Saunders A.M., Hulette C., Welsh-Bohmer K.A., Schmechel D.E., et al. Specificity, sensitivity and predictive value of apolipoprotein-E genotyping for sporadic Alzheimer's disease. Lancet 1993 Jul; 348: 90.

Shin R.W., Lee V.M., Trojanowski J.Q. Neurofibrillary pathology and aluminum in Alzheimer's disease. Histol Histopathol 1995 Oct; 10(4): 969–78.

Singh V.K. Studies of neuroimmune markers in Alzheimer's disease. Mol Neurobiol 1994 Aug-Dec; 9(1–3): 73–81.

Sisodia S.S., Koo E.H., Beyreuther K., Unterbeck A., Price D.L. Evidence that B-amyloid protein in Alzheimer's disease is not derived by normal processing. Science 1990; 248: 492–5.

Soderberg M., Edlund C., Kristensson K., Dallner G. The fatty acid composition of brain phospholipids in aging and in Alzheimer's disease. Lipids 1991 Jun; 26(6): 421–5.

Spagnoli A., et al. Long-term acetyl-L-carnitine treatment in Alzheimer's disease. Neurology 1991 Nov; 41: 1726–32.

Steventon G.B., et al. Xenobiotic metabolism in Alzheimer's disease. Neurology 1990 Jul; 40: 1095–8.

Stoll S., Scheuer K., Pohl O., Muller W.E. Ginkgo biloba extract (EGb 761) independently improves changes in passive avoidance learning and brain membrane fluidity in the aging mouse. Pharmacopsychiat 1996 Jul; 29(4): 144–9.

Svec F. and Lopez A. Antiglucocorticoid actions of dehydroepiandrosterone and low concentrations in Alzheimer's disease. Lancet 1989 Dec 2: 1335–6.

Taylor G.A., et al. Gastrointestinal absorption of aluminum in Alzheimer's disease: response to aluminum citrate. Age and Aging 1992; 21: 81–90.

Thal L.J., et al. A one-year, multicenter placebo controlled study of ALC in patients with Alzheimer's. Neurology 1996; 477: 705–11.

Volicer L., Crino P.B., et al. Involvement of free radicals in dementia of the Alzheimer type: a hypothesis. Neurobiol of Aging 1990; 11: 567–71.

Williams A. Alzheimer's disease and nutrition. British J of Hospital Med 1991 Jan; 45: 12.

Winograd C.H., et al. Nutritional intake in patients with senile dementia of the Alzheimer's type. Alzheimer's Disease and Associated Disorders 1991; 5(3): 173–80.

Yankner B.A. and Mesulam M. B-amyloid and the pathogenesis of Alzheimer's disease. N Engl J Med 1991 Dec. 26; 325(26): 1849–57.

Yokel R.A. Aluminum exposure produces learning and memory deficits: a model of Alzheimer's disease. In Toxin-Induced Models of Neurologic Disorders, Woodruff, M.I. and Nonneman A., eds. Penum Press 1994, Chap. 11; 301–18.

Yokoyama H., Lingle D.M., Crestranello J.A., et al. Coenzyme Q10 protects coronary endothelial function from ischemia reperfusion injury via an antioxidant effect. Surgery 1996 Aug; 120(2): 189–96.

Zhou Y., Richardson J.S., Mombourquette M.J., Weil J.A. Free radical formation in autopsy samples of Alzheimer and control cortex. Neurotoxic Lett 1995 Aug 4; 195(2): 89–92.

Zubenko G.S., Wusylko M., Cohen B.M., Boller F., Telpy I. Family study of platelet membrane fluidity in Alzheimer's disease. Science 1987; 238: 539–42.

• Chapter Six: Parkinson's Disease

Abbott R.A., Cox M., Markus H., Tomkins A. Diet, body size and micronutrient status in Parkinson's disease. Eur J Clin Nutr 1992 Dec; 46(12): 879–84.

Adams J.D., Klaidman L.K., Odunze I.N., et al. Alzheimer's and

Parkinson's diseases. Brain levels of glutathione, glutathione disulfide, and vitamin E. Biol Chem Nueropathol 1991 Jun; 14(3): 213–2.

Astarloa R., Mena M.A., Sanchez V., et al. Clinical and pharmacokinetic effects of a diet rich in insoluble fiber on Parkinson's disease. Clin Neuropharmacol 1992 Oct; 15(5): 375–80.

Beal M.F. Aging, energy, and oxidative stress in neurodegenerative diseases. Ann Neurol 1995; 38: 357–66.

Beal M.F. Does impairment of energy metabolism result in excitotoxic neuronal death in neurodegenerative illnesses? Ann Neurol 1992; 31: 119–30.

Beuter A., Mergler D., de Geoffroy A., et al. Diadochokinesimetry: a study of patients with Parkinson's disease and manganese exposed workers. NeuroToxicology 1994 Fall; 15(3): 655–64.

Birkmayer J.G., Vrecko C., Volc D., Birkmayer W. Nicotinamide adenine dinucleotide (NADH)—a new therapeutic approach to Parkinson's disease. Acta Neurol Scand 1993; 87: Suppl 146: 32–5.

Birkmayer W. and Birkmayer G.J.D. Strategic and tactic of modern Parkinson therapy. Acta Neurol Scand 1989; 126: 63–6.

Burkhardt C.R. and Weber H.K. Parkinson's disease: a chronic, low-grade antioxidant deficiency? Med Hypotheses 1994 Aug; 43(2): 111–4.

Cabrera-Valdivia F., Jimenez-Jimenez F.J., Molina J.A., et al. Peripheral iron metabolism in patients with Parkinson's disease. J Neurol Sci 1994 Aug; 125(1): 82–6.

Carter J.H., Nutt J.G., Woodward W.F., et al. Amount and distribution of dietary protein affects clinical response to levodopa in Parkinson's disease. Neurology 1989 Apr; 39(4): 552–6.

Carvey P.M., et al. The potent use of a dopamine neuron antibody and a striatal neurotrophic factor as diagnostic markers in Parkinson's. Neurology 1995; 41: S3–8.

Croxson S., et al. Dietary modification of Parkinson's disease. Eur J of Clin Nut 1991; 45: 263–6.

Dexter D.T., Carayon A., Javoy-Agid F., et al. Alterations in the levels of iron, ferritin and other trace metals in Parkinson's disease and other neurodegenerative diseases affecting the basal ganglia. Brain 1991; 114: 1953–75.

Dizdar N., Kagedal B., Lindvall B. Treatment of Parkinson's disease with NADH. Acta Neurol Scand 1994 Nov; 90(5): 345–7.

Fahn S. An open trial of high-dose antioxidants in early Parkinson's disease. Am J of Clin Nut 1991; 53: 380S–382S.

Gimenez-Roldan S. and Mateo D. Predicting beneficial response to a protein-redistribution diet in fluctuating in Parkinson's disease. Acta Neurol Bel 1991; 91(4): 189–200.

Gimenez-Roldan S., Mateo D., Garcia A.A., Garcia P.P. Proposal for a protein redistribution diet in the control of motor fluctuations in Parkinson's disease: acceptance and efficacy. Neurologia 1991 Jan; 6(1): 3–9.

Gorell J.M., et al. Increased iron-related MRI contrast in the substantia nigra in Parkinson's disease. Neurol 1995 Jun; 45(6): 1138–43.

Griffiths P.D. and Crossman A.R. Distribution of iron in the basal ganglia and neocortex in postmortem tissue in Parkinson's disease and Alzheimer's disease. Dementia 1993 Mar-Apr; 4(2): 61–5.

Grimes J.D., Hassan M.N., Thakar J. Antioxidant therapy in Parkinson's disease. Can J Neurol Sci 1987 Aug; 14(3 Suppl): 483–7.

Hantraye P., Brouillet E., Ferrante R., Palfi S., et al. Inhibition of neuronal nitric oxide synthase prevents MPTP-induced parkinsonism in baboons. Nature Medicine 1996 Sept; 2(9): 1017.

Harley Al, Cooper J.M., Schapira A.H. Iron induced oxidative stress and mitochondrial dysfunction: relevance to Parkinson's disease. Brain Res 1993 Nov 12; 627(2): 349–53.

Jellinger K.A., Kienzl E., Rumpelmaier G., et al. Iron and ferritin in substantia nigra in Parkinson's disease. Adv Neurol 1993; 60: 267–72.

Jener P. Altered mitochondrial function, iron metabolism and glutathione levels in Parkinson's disease. Acta Nuerol Scand Suppl 1993; 146: 6–13.

Jimenez-Jimenez F.J., Molina J.A., Aguilar M.V., et al. Serum and urinary manganese levels in patients with Parkinson's disease. Acta Neurol Scand 1995 May; 91(5): 317–20.

Kalra J., Rajput A.H., Mantha S.V., Prasad K. Serum antioxidant enzyme activity in Parkinson's disease. Mol Cell Biochem 1992 Mar 25; 110(2): 165–8.

Karstaedt P.J. and Pincus J.H. Protein redistribution diet remains effective in patients with fluctuating parkinsonism. Arch Neurol 1992 Feb; 49: 149–51.

Karstaedt P.J., Pincus J.H., Coughlin S.S. Standard and controlled-release levodopa/carbidopa in patients with fluctuating Parkinson's disease on a protein redistribution diet. A preliminary report. Arch Neurol 1991 Apr; 48(4): 402–5.

Koller W., Vetere-Overfield B., Gray C., et al. Environmental risk factors in Parkinson's disease. Neurology 1990 Aug; 40: 1218–21.

Lichter D., Kurlan R., Miller C., Shoulson I. Does pergolide slow the progression of Parkinson's disease? A 7-year follow-up study. Neurology 1988 Mar; 38(Suppl 1): 122.

Loeffler D.A., Connor J.R., Juneau P.L., et al. Transferrin and iron in normal, Alzheimer's disease, and Parkinson's disease brain regions. J Neurochem 1995 Aug; 65(2): 710–24.

Mann V.M., Cooper J.M., Daniel S.E., et al. Complex I, iron, and ferritin in Parkinson's disease substantia nigra. Ann Neurol 1994 Dec; 36(6): 876–81.

Meister A. Mitochondrial changes associated with glutathione deficiency. Biochim et Biophys Acta 1995; 1271: 35–42.

Mizuno Y., Ikebe S., Hattori N., et al. Role of mitochondria in the etiology and pathogenesis of Parkinson's disease. Biochim Biophys Acta 1995 May 24; 1271(1): 265–74.

Mizuno Y., Shin-ichirou I., Nobutaka H., et al. Role of mitochondria in the etiology and pathogenesis of Parkinson's disease Biochim et Biophys Acta 1995; 1271: 265–74.

Mohr E., et al. Neuropsychological and glucose metabolic profiles in asymmetric Parkinson's disease. Can J of Neurol Sci 1992; 19: 163–9.

Monte D., et al. Glutathione in Parkinson's disease: a link between oxidative stress and mitochondrial damage. Ann Neurol 1992; 32: S111–S15.

Montgomery E.B. Heavy metals and the etiology of Parkinson's disease and other movement disorders. Toxicology 1995 Mar 31; 97(1–3): 3–9.

Morris C.M. and Edwardson J.A. Iron histochemistry of the substantia nigra in Parkinson's disease. Neurodegeneration 1994 Dec; 3(4): 277–82.

Nutt J.G. and Carter J.H. Therapy of Parkinson's disease and diet issues in the treatment of Parkinson's disease. In Therapy of Parkinson's Disease, Elsevier Science Inc. 1990, Chapter 28.

Olanow C.W. An introduction to the free radical hypothesis in Parkinson's disease. Ann Neurol 1992; 32: S2–S9.

Olanow C.W., et al. The effect of deprenyl and levodopa on the progression of Parkinson's. Ann Neurol 95; 38: 71–8.

The Parkinson Study Group. Effect of deprenyl on the progression of disability in early Parkinson's disease. N Engl J Med 1989 Nov 16; 321(20): 1364–71.

The Parkinson Study Group. Effects of tocopherol and deprenyl on the progression of disability in early Parkinson's disease. N Engl J Med 1993 Jan 21; 328(3): 176–83.

Peppard R.F., et al. Cerebral glucose metabolism in Parkinson's disease with and without dementia. Arch Neurol 1992 Dec; 49: 1262–8.

Riley D. and Lang A.E. Practical application of a low-protein diet for Parkinson's disease. Neurol 1988 Jul; 38(7); 1026–31.

Sanchis G., Mena M.A., Martin del Rio R., et al. Effect of a controlled low-protein diet on the pharmacological response to levodopa and on the plasma levels of L-dopa and amino acids in patients with Parkinson's disease. Arch Neurobiol 1991 Nov-Dec; 54(6): 296–302.

Schapira A.H. Evidence for mitochondrial dysfunction in Parkinson's disease—a critical appraisal. Mov Disord 1994 Mar; 9(2): 125–38.

Schapira A.H.V., Cooper J.M., Dexter D., Clark J.B., Jenner P., Marsden C.D. Mitochondrial complex I deficiency in Parkinson's disease. J of Neurochem 1990; 54(3): 823–7.

Schapira A.H., Hartley A., Cleeter M.W., Cooper J.M. Free radicals and mitochondrial dysfunction in Parkinson's disease. Biochem Soc Trans 1993 May; 21(2): 367–70.

Schulz J.B., Henshaw D.R., Matthews R.T., Beal M.F. Coenzyme Q10 and nicotinamide: a free radical spin trap protect against MPTP neurotoxicity. Experimental Neurol 1995; 135(2): 279–83.

Sian J., Dexter D.T., Lees A.J., et al. Alterations in glutathione levels in Parkinson's disease and other neurodegenerative disorders affecting basal ganglia. Ann Neurol 1994; 36: 348–55.

Singer T.P., Ramsay R.R., Ackresll B.A. Efficiencies of NADH and succinate dehydrogenases in degenerative diseases and myopathies. Biochim Biophys Acta (Netherlands) 1995 May 24; 1271 (1): 211–9.

Snyder S.H. No NO prevents parkinsonism. Nature Medicine 1996 Sept; 2(9): 965–6.

Stevenson G.B., et. al. Xenobiotic metabolism in Parkinson's disease. Neurology 1989; 883–7.

Tanner, C.M. Liver enzyme abnormalities in Parkinson's disease. Geriatrics 1991 Aug; 46 (Suppl 1): 60–3.

Tanner C.M. and Langston J.W. Do environmental toxins cause Parkinson's disease? A critical review. Neurology 1990; 40 (Suppl 3): 17–30.

Taylor D.J., Drige D., Barnes P.R., Kemp G.J., et al. A 31P magnetic resonance spectroscopy study of mitochondrial function in skeletal muscle of patients with Parkinson's disease. J Neurol Sci 1994 Aug; 125(1): 77–81.

Tetrud J.W. and Langston J.W. The effect of deprenyl (selegiline) on the natural history of Parkinson's disease. Science 1989 Aug; 4: 519–22.

Vatassery G.T. Vitamin E neurochemistry and implications for neurodegeneration in Parkinson's disease. Ann NY Acad Sci 1992 Sept 30; 669: 97–109.

Vieregge P., et al. Lifestyle and dietary factors early and late in Parkinson's disease. Can J of Neurol Sci 1992; 19 (2): 170–3.

Yasui M., et al. Calcium, magnesium and aluminum concentrations in Parkinson's disease. NeuroToxicology 1992; 13: 593–6.

Youdim M. New perspectives in nutritional therapies. Ann NY Acad Sci 1994; 738: 64–7.

Youdim M.B., Ben-Shachar D., Eshel G., et al. The neurotoxicity of iron and nitric oxide. Relevance to the etiology of Parkinson's disease. Adv Neurol 1993; 60: 259–66.

Youdim M.B., Ben-Shachar D., Riederer P. The possible role of iron in the etiopathology of Parkinson's disease. Mov Disord 1993; 8(1): 1–12.

Youdim M.B. and Riederer P. The role of iron in senescence of dopaminergic neurons in Parkinson's disease. J Neural Transm 1993; 40 (Suppl): 57–67.

### • Chapter Seven: Multiple Sclerosis

Aberg J.A., et al. Prostaglandin production in chronic progressive mutiple sclerosis. J of Clin Lab Analysis 1990; 4: 246–50.

Ansari K.A. and Shoeman D.W. Arachidonic and docosahexanoic acid content of bovine brain myelin: implications for the pathogenesis of multiple sclerosis. Neurochem Res 1990 Jan; 15(1): 7–11.

Bates D., Cartlidge N.E.F., French J.M., et al. A double-blind controlled trial of long chain n–3 polyunsaturated fatty acids in the treatment of multiple sclerosis. Journal of Neurology, Neurosurgery, and Psychiatry 1989; 52: 18–22.

Beck W. Megaloblastic anemias. Cecil Textbook of Medicine. Wyngarden and Smith, eds. 17th ed., W.B. Saunders, 1985.

Ben-Shlomo Y., Davey S.G., Marmot M.G. Dietary fat in the epidemiology of multiple sclerosis; has the situation been adequately assessed? Neuroepidemiology 1992; 11 (4–6): 214–25.

Boullerne A.I., Petry K.G., Geffard M. Circulating antibodies directed against conjugated fatty acids in sera of patients with multiple sclerosis. J Neuroimmunol 1996; 65: 75–81.

Bray P.F., Luka J., Bray P.F., Culp K.W., Schlight J.P. Antibodies against Epstein-Barr nuclear antigen (EBNA) in multiple sclerosis CSF, and two pentapeptide sequence identities between EBNA any myelin basic protein. Neurology 1992; 42: 1798–1804.

Chelmicka-Schorr E. and Aranson B.G. Nervous system–immune system interactions and their role in multiple sclerosis. Ann Neurol 1994; 36: S29–S32.

Fitzgerald G., Harbige L.S., Forti A., Crawford M.A. The effect of nutritional counselling on diet and plasma EFA status in multiple sclerosis patients over 3 years. Hum Nutr Appl Nutr 1987 Oct; 41(5): 297–310.

Frequin S.T., Wevers R.A., Braam M., et al. Decreased vitamin B12 and folate levels in cerebrospinal fluid and serum of multiple sclerosis patients after high-dose intravenous methylprednisolone. J Neurol 1993 May; 240(5): 305–8.

Goldberg P., Fleming M.C., Picard E.H. Multiple sclerosis: decreased relapse rate through dietary supplementation with calcium, magnesium and vitamin D. Med Hypotheses 1986 Oct; 21 (2): 193–200.

Goodkin D.E., Jacobsen D.W., Green R. Biologically significant serum vitamin B12 deficiency in multiple sclerosis inadequately documented. Arch Neurol 1992 Jul; 49 (7): 683–4.

Grasso G. and Muscettola M. Possible role of gamma interferon in ovarian function. Ontogenetic and Phylogenetic Mechanisms of Neuroimmunomodulation. Fabris N., Jankovic B., Markovic B. and Spector N., eds. Ann NY Acad Sci 1992; Vol. 650.

Gruener D.M., Kunkel E.J., Snyderman D.A., et al. Dietary vitamin B12 deficiency in a patient with multiple sclerosis. Gen Hosp Psychiatry 1994 May; 16 (3): 224–8.

Hauser S., et al. Antispacticity effect of threonine in MS. Arch Neurol 1992 Sept; 49: 923–6.

Holman R.T., Johnson S.B., Kokmen E. Deficiencies of polyunsaturated fatty acids and replacement by nonessential fatty acids in plasma lipids in multiple sclerosis. Proc Natl Acad Sci 1989 Jun; 86: 4720–4.

Hutter C.D. and Laing P. Multiple sclerosis: sunlight, diet, immunology and aetiology. Med Hypotheses 1996 Feb; 46 (2): 67–74.

Jacobs L.D., et al. Intramuscular interferon beta 1-A for disease progression in relapsing multiple sclerosis. Ann Neurol 1996; 39: 285–94.

Johnson K.P. Experimental therapy of relapsing-remitting multiple sclerosis with copolymer-1. Ann Neurol 1994; 36: S115–17.

Johnson K.P., Brooks B.R., Cohen J.A., et al. Copolymer 1 reduces relapse rate and improves disability in relapsing-remitting multiple sclerosis: results of a phase III multicenter, double-blind, placebo-controlled trial. Neurology 1995 Jul; 45: 1268–75.

Kira J., Tobimatsu S., Goto I. Vitamin B12 metabolism and massive-dose methyl vitamin B12 in Japanese patients with multiple sclerosis. Intern Med 1994 Feb; 33 (2): 82–6.

Kruger P.G. and Nyland H.I. The role of mast cells and diet in the onset and maintenance of multiple sclerosis: a hypothesis. Med Hypotheses 1995 Jan; 44 (1): 66–9.

Lehmann D., Karussis D., Misrachi-Koll R., et al. Oral adminstration of the oxidant-scavenger N-acetyl-L-cysteine inhibits acute experimental autoimmune encephalomyelitis. J Neuroimmunol 1994; 50: 35–42.

Logigian E.L., Kaplan R.F., Steere A.C. Chronic neurologic manifestations of Lyme disease. N Engl J Med 1990 Nov 22; 323 (21): 1438–44.

Mai J., et al. High dose antioxidant supplementation to MS patients: effects on glutathione peroxidase, clinical safety, and absorption of selenium. Biol Trace Element Res 1990; 24: 109–17.

Manley P. Diet in multiple sclerosis. Practitioner 1994 May; 238 (1538): 358–63.

Monastra G., Cross A.H., Bruni A., Raine C.S. Phosphatidylserine, a putative inhibitor of tumor necrosis factor, prevents autoimmune demyelination. Neurology 1993 Jan; 43: 153–62.

Neu I., et al. Leukotrienes in the cerebrospinal fluid of multiple sclerosis patients. Acta Neurol Scand 1992; 86: 586–7.

Nieves J., Cosman F., Herbert J., et al. High prevalence of vitamin D deficiency and reduced bone mass in multiple sclerosis. Neurology 1994 Sept; 44 (9): 1687–92.

Nightingale S., Woo E., Smith A.D., et al. Red blood cell and adipose tissue fatty acids in mild inactive multiple sclerosis. Acta Neurol Scand 1990; 82: 43–50.

Nijst T.Q., Wevers R.A., Schoonderwaldt H.C., et al. Vitamin B12 and folate concentrations in serum and cerebrospinal fluid of neurological patients with special reference to multiple sclerosis and dementia. J Neurol Neurosurg Psychiatry 1990 Nov; 53 (11): 951–4.

Reynolds E.H. Multiple sclerosis and vitamin B12 metabolism. J Neuroimmunol 1992 Oct; 40 (2–3): 225–30.

Reynolds E.H. Multiple sclerosis and vitamin B12 metabolism. J Neurol Neurosurg Psychiatry 1992 May; 55 (5): 339–40.

Reynolds E.H., Bottigliere T., Laundy M., et al. Vitamin B12 metabolism in multiple sclerosis. Arch Neurol 1992 Jun; 49 (6): 649–52.

Reynolds E.H., Linnell J.C., Faludy J.E. Multiple sclerosis associated with vitamin B12 deficiency. Arch Neurol 1991 Aug; 48 (8): 808–11.

Rieckmann P., Albrecht M., Kitze B., Weber T., et al. Tumor necrosis factor-alpha messenger RNA expression in patients with relapsing-remitting multiple sclerosis is associated with disease activity. Ann Neurol 1995 Jan; 37 (1): 82–88.

Robinson M.K. Glutathione deficiency and HIV infection. Lancet 1992 Jun 27; 339: 1603–4.

Sandyk R. and Awerbuch G.I. Vitamin B12 and its relationship to age of onset of multiple sclerosis. Int J Neurosci 1993 Jul-Aug; 71 (1–4): 93–9.

Schwartz G.G. Hypothesis: calcitriol mediates pregnancy's protective effect on multiple sclerosis. Arch Neurol May 1993; 50: 455.

Sharief M.K. and Hentges R. Association between tumor necrosis factor-alpha and disease progression in patients with multiple sclerosis. N Engl J Med 1991 Aug 15; 325 (7): 467–71.

Sharief M.K., Noori M.A., Ciardi M., Cirelli A., Thompson E.J. Increased levels of circulating ICAM-1 in serum and cerebrospinal fluid of patients with active multiple sclerosis. Correlation with TNF-alpha and blood-brain barrier damage. J Neuroimmunol 1993 Mar; 43 (1–2): 15–21.

Steinman L. Autoimmune disease: misguided assaults on the self produce multiple sclerosis, juvenile diabetes and other chronic illnesses. Promising therapies are emerging. Scientific American 1993 Sept: 107–14.

Sumaya C.V., Myers L.W., Ellison G.W., Ench Y. Increased prevalence and titer of Epstein-Barr virus antibodies in patients with multiple sclerosis. Ann Neurol 1985; 17: 371–77.

Swank R.L. Multiple sclerosis; fat-oil relationship. Nutrition 1991 Sept-Oct; 7 (5): 368–76.

Swank R.L. and Dugan B.B. Effect of low saturated fat diet in early and late causes of multiple sclerosis. Lancet 1990 Jul 7; 336 (8706): 37–9.

Toshniwal P. and Zarling E. Increased free radicals in multiple sclerosis. Neurochem Res 1992; 17: 207–7.

Wong E.K., Enomoto H., Leopold I.H., et al. Intestinal absorption of dietary fat in patients with multiple sclerosis. Metab Pediatr Syst Ophthalmol 1993; 16 (3–4): 39–42.

Yasui M., et al. Magnesium concentration in brains from multiple sclerosis patients. Acta Neurol Scand 1990; 81: 197–200.

Yoon C.K. MS study yields mixed results. Science 1993 Feb; 259: 1263.

• *Chapter Eight: Amyotrophic Lateral Sclerosis*

Aschner M. Methylmercury in astrocytes—what possible significance? NeuroToxicology 1996; 17 (1): 93–106.

Ashmead, H.D. Increased superoxide dismutase activity resulting from ingested amino acid chelated minerals. Paper presented at Albion Laboratories International Conference on Human Nutrition, Salt Lake City, Utah, Jan 21–22, 1995.

Barrett-Connor E., Khaw K.T., Yen S.S.C. Prospective study of dehydroepiandrosterone sulfate, mortality, and cardiovascular disease. N Engl J Med 1986 Dec 11; 315 (24): 1519–24.

Beckman J.S., Carson M., Smith C.D., Koppenol W.H. ALS, SOD and peroxynitrite (letter). Nature 1993 Aug 12; 364 (6438): 584.

Bensimon G., Lacomblez L., Meininger, and the ALS/Riluzole Study Group. A controlled trial of riluzole in amyotrophic lateral sclerosis. N Engl J Med 1994 Mar 3; 330 (9): 585–91.

Bergeron C., Muntasser S., Somerville M.J., Weyer L., Percy M.E. Copper/zinc superoxide dismutase mRNA levels are increased in sporadic amyotrophic lateral sclerosis motor neurons. Brain Res 1994 Oct 3; 659 (1–2): 272–6.

Bologa L., Sharma J., Roberts E. Dehydroepiandrosterone and its sulfated derivative reduce neuronal death and enhance astrocytic differentiation in brain cultures. J of Neuroscience Res 1987; 17: 225–34.

Bowling A.C., Schulz J.B., Brown R.H., Beal M.F. Superoxide dismutase activity, oxidative damage, and mitochondrial energy metabolism in familial and sporadic amyotrophic lateral sclerosis. J Neurochem 1993 Dec; 61 (6): 2322–5.

Bristol L.A., Rothstein J.D. Glutamate transporter gene expression in amyotrophic lateral sclerosis motor cortex. Ann Neurol 1996 May; 39: 676–9.

Brooks N. In vitro evidence for a role of glutamate in CNS toxicity of mercury. Toxicology 1992; 76: 245–6.

Chaudhry V., Corse A.M., Cornblath D.R., et al. Multifocal motor neuropathy: response to human immune globulin. Ann Neurol 1993 Mar; 33 (3): 237–42.

Choi D.W. Methods for antagonizing glutamate neurotoxicity. Cerebrovascular and Brain Metabolism Rev 1990; 2: 105–47.

Colasanti M., Persichini T., Menegazzi M., et al. Introduction of nitric oxide synthase mRNA expression. Suppression by exogenous nitric oxide. J Biol Chem 1995 Nov 10; 270 (45): 26731–3.

Darley-Usmar V., Wiseman H., Halliwell B. Nitric oxide and oxygen radicals: a question of balance. FEBS Lett 1995 Aug 7; 369 (2–3): 131–5.

Dawsen T.M., et al. The immunosuppressant FK506 enhances phosphaphoralation of nitric oxide synthase and protects against glutamate neurotoxicity. Proc Nat Acad Sci 1993; 90: 9808–12.

Dawsen T.M., et al. Mechanisms of nitric oxide mediated neurotoxicity in primary brain cultures. J Neurosci 1993; 13: 2651–61.

DiSilvestro, R.T., et al. Effects of copper supplementation on ceruloplasmin and copper-zinc superoxide dismutase in free-living rheumatoid arthritis patients. J Am Coll Nutr 1992; 11: 177.

Eisen A., Pearmain J., Stewart H. Dehydroepiandrosterone sulphate (DHEAS) concentrations and amyotrophic lateral sclerosis. Muscle & Nerv 1995 Dec; 18: 1481–1483.

Fagni L., Lafon-Cazal M., Lerner-Natoli M., et al. J Pharm Belg 1995 Mar-Jun; 50 (2–3): 204–12.

Festoff B.W., Yang S.X., Vaught J., Bryan C., Ma J.Y. J Neurol Sci 1995 May; 129: S114–S121.

Fisman, M. Hepatic ultrastructural change and liver dysfunction in amyotrophic lateral sclerosis. Arch Neurol 1987 Oct; 44 (10): 103–6.

Garafolo O., et al. Superoxide dismutase activity in lymphoblastoid cells from motor neuron disease/amyotrophic lateral sclerosis (MND/ALS) patients. J Neurol Sci 1995 May; 129 (Suppl): 90–2.

Gredal O. and Moller S.E. Effect of branched-chain amino acids on glutamate metabolism in amyotrophic lateral sclerosis. J Neurol Sci 1995 Mar; 129 (1): 40–3.

Greenhaff P.L., Bodin K., Soderlund K., Hultman E. The effect of oral creatine supplementation on skeletal muscle phosphocreatine resynthesis. Am J Physiol 1994; 266: E725–E730.

Greenhaff P.L., Casey A., Short A.H., et al. Influence of oral creatine supplementation of muscle torque during repeated bouts of maximal voluntary exercise in man. Clin Sci 1993; 84: 565–71.

Gurney M.E., Cutting F.B., Zhai P., Doble A., et al. Benefit of vitamin E, riluzole, and gabapentin in a transgenic model of familial amyotrophic lateral sclerosis. Ann Neurol 1996 Fed; 39 (2): 147–57.

Harris R.C., Soderlund K., Hultman E. Elevation of creatine in resting and exercised muscle of normal subjects by creatine supplementation. Clin Sci 1992; 83: 367–74.

Ihara Y., Mori A., Hayabara T., Kawai M., et al. Superoxide dismutase and free radicals in sporadic amyotrophic lateral sclerosis:

relationship to clinical data. J Neurol Sci 1995 Dec; 134 (1–2): 51–6.

Ikeda K., Linkosz B., Greene T., et al. Effects of brain-derived neurotropic factor on motor dysfunction in wobbler mouse motor neuron disease. Ann Neurol 1995 Apr; 37 (4): 505–11.

The Italian Study Group. Branched-chain amino acids and amyotrophic lateral sclerosis: a treatment failure? Neurology 1993 Dec; 43 (12): 2466–70. Comment in: Neurology 1993 Dec; 43 (12): 2437–8.

Kasarskis E.J., Tandon L., Lovell M.A., Ehmann W.D. Aluminum, calcium and iron in the spinal cords of patients with sporadic amyotrophic lateral sclerosis using laser microprobe mass spectroscopy: a preliminary study. J Neurol Sci 1995 Jun; 130 (2): 203–8.

Lang D.J. Recombinant human insulin-like growth factors in ALS. Neurol 1996; 47: S93–5.

Lindsay R.M. Trophic protection of motor neurons: clinical potential in motor neuron diseases. J Neurol 1994 Dec; 242 (Suppl 1): S8–S11.

Lipton S.A. and Rosenberg P.A. Excitatory amino acids as a final common pathway for neurologic disorders. N Engl J Med 1994 Mar 3; 330 (9): 613–22.

Louwerse E.S., Buchet J.P., Van Diijik M.A., et al. Urinary excretion of lead and mercury after oral administration of meso-2, 3-dimercaptosuccinic acid in patients with motor neuron disease. Int Arch Occup Environ Health 1995; 67 (2): 135–8.

Louwerse E.S., Weverling G.J., Bossuyt P.M., Meyjes F.E., de Jong J.M. Randomized, double-blind, controlled trial of acetylcysteine in amyotrophic lateral sclerosis. Arch Neurol 1995 Jun; 52 (6): 559–64.

Lipton S.A. and Rosenberg, P.A. Excitatory amino acids as a final common pathway for neurologic disorders. N Engl J Med 1994 Mar 3; 330 (9): 613–22.

Lyons T.J., Liu H., Goto J.J., Nersissian A. et al. Mutations in copper-zinc superoxide dismutase that cause amyotrophic lateral sclerosis alter the zinc binding site and the redox behavior of the protein. Proc Natl Acad Sci 1996 Oct 29; 93 (22): 12240–4.

Malessa S., Leigh P.N., Bertel O., Sluga E., Hornykiewicz O. Amyotrophic lateral sclerosis: glutamate dehydrogenase and transmitter amino acids in the spinal cord. J Neurol Neurosurg Psychiatry 1991 Nov; 54 (11): 984–8.

Marx J. Gene linked to Lou Gehrig's disease. Science 1993 Mar 5; 259 (5100): 1393.

McNamara J.O. and Fridovich, I. Did radicals strike Lou Gehrig? Nature 1993 Mar 4; 362: 20–1.

Mitani K. Relationship between neurological diseases due to aluminum load, especially amyotrophic lateral sclerosis, and magnesium status. Magnes Res 1992 Sept.; 5 (3): 203–13.

Morales A.J., Nolan J.J., Nelson J.C., Yen S.S. Effects of replacement dose of dehydroepiandrosterone in men and women of advancing age. J Clin Endocrinol Metab 1994 Jun; 78 (6): 1360–7.

Moriwaka F., Satoh H., Ejima A., Watanabe E. et al. Mercury and selenium contents in amyotrophic lateral sclerosis in Hokkaido, the northernmost island of Japan. J Neurol Sci 1993 Aug; 118 (1): 38–42.

Nakano Y., Hirayama K., Terao K. Hepatic ultrastructural changes and liver dysfunction in amyotrophic lateral sclerosis. Arch Neurol 1987 Jan; 44 (1): 103–6.

Nishida C.R., Gralla E.B., Valengine J.S. Characterization of three yeast copper-zinc superoxide dismutase mutants analogous to those coded for in familial amyotrophic lateral sclerosis. Proc Natl Acad Sci 1994 Oct 11; 91 (21): 9906–10.

Paakkari I. and Lindsberg P. Nitric oxide in the central nervous system. Ann Med 1995 Jun; 27 (3): 369–77.

Park S.T., Lim K.T., Chung, Y.T., Kim S.U. Methylmercury-induced neurotoxicity in cerebral neuron culture is blocked by antioxidants and NMDA receptor antagonists. NeuroToxicology 1996; 17 (1): 37–46.

Pestronk A., Adams R.N., Clawson L., et al. Serum antibodies to GM1 ganglioside in amyotrophic lateral sclerosis. Neurology 1988; 38: 1457–61.

Piccardo P., Yanagiahara R., Garruto R.M., Gibbs C.J., Gajdusek D.C. Histochemical and x-ray microanalytical localization of aluminum in amyotrophic lateral sclerosis and parkinsonism-dementia of Guam. Acta Neuropathol 1988; 77 (1): 1–4.

Plaitikis A. and Carascio J.T. Abnormal glutamate metabolism in ALS. Ann Neurol 1987; 22: 5755–9.

Plaitakis A. and Constantakakis E. Altered metabolism of excitatory amino acids, n-acetyl-aspartate and n-acetyl-aspartyl-glutamate in amyotrophic lateral sclerosis. Brain Res Bull 1993; 30 (3–4): 381–6.

Plaitakis A., Constantakakis E., Smith J. The neuroexcitoxic amino acids glutamate and aspartate are altered in the spinal cord and brain in amyotrophic lateral sclerosis. Ann Neurol 1988 Sept.; 24 (3): 446–9.

Postam C.T., Hoefnagels W.H.L., Thien Th., DeBoo Th. Zinc, glutamate receptors, and motorneurone disease. Lancet 1987 Nov 7: 1082–84.

Przedborski, S., et al. Brain superoxide dismutase, catalase, and glutathione peroxidase activities in amyotrophic lateral sclerosis. Ann Neurol 1996; 39 (2): 158–65.

Ratan R.R., Murphy T.H., Baraban J.M. Macromolecular synthesis inhibitors prevent oxidative stress-induced apoptosis in embryonic cortical neurons by shunting cysteine from protein synthesis to glutathione. J Neuroscience 1994 Jul; 14 (7): 4385–92.

Reiner A., Medina L., Figueredo-Cardenas G., Anfinson S. Brainstem motoneuron pools that are selectively resistant in amyotrophic lateral sclerosis are preferentially enriched in parvalbumin: evidence from monkey brainstem for a calcium-mediated mechanism in sporadic ALS. Exp Neurol 1995 Feb; 131 (2): 239–50.

Rosen D.R., Siddique T., Patterson D., et al. Mutations in Cu/Zn superoxide dismutase gene are associated with familial amyotrophic lateral sclerosis. Nature 1993 Mar 4; 362: 59–62.

Rothstein J.D., Bristol L.A., Hosler B., Brown R.H., Kunci R.W. Chronic inhibition of superoxide dismutase produces apoptotic death of spinal neurons. Proc Natl Acad Sci 1994 May; 91: 4155–59.

Rothstein J.D. and Kunch R.W. Neuroprotective strategies in a model of chronic glutamate-mediated motor neuron toxicity, J Neurochem 1995 Aug; 65 (2): 643–51.

Rothstein J.D., Martin L.J., Kunch R.W. Decreased glutamate transport by the brain and spinal cord in amyotrophic lateral sclerosis. N Engl J Med 1992 May 28; 326 (22): 1464–95.

Rowland L.P. Amyotrophic lateral sclerosis. Cur Opin Neurol 1994 Aug; 7 (4): 310–15.

Sarafian T.A., Bredesen D.E., Verity M.A. Cellular resistance to methylmercury. NeuroToxicology 1996; 17 (1): 27–36.

Seeburger J.L. and Springer J.E. Experimental rationale for the therapeutic use of neurotrophins in amyotrophic lateral sclerosis. Exp Neurol 1993 Nov; 124 (1): 64–72.

Smith R.G. and Appel S.H. Molecular approaches to amyotrophic lateral sclerosis. Ann Rev Med 1995; 46: 133–45.

Szerb J.C. and O'Regan P.A. Glutamine enhances glutamate release in preference to gamma-aminobutyrate release in hippocampal slices. Can J Physiol Pharmcol 1984 Aug; 62 (8): 919–23.

Testa D., Carceni T., Fetoni V. Branched-chain amino acids in the treatment of amyotrophic lateral sclerosis. J Neurol 1989 Dec; 236 (8): 445–7.

Uchino M., Ando Y., Tanaka Y., Nakamura T., et al. Decrease in Cu/Zn- and Mn-superoxide dismutase activities in brain and spinal cord of patients with amyotrophic lateral sclerosis. J Neurol Sci 1994 Dec 1; 127 (1): 61–7.

Wakai M.,Mokuno K., Hashizume Y., Kato K. An immunohistochemical study of the neuronal expression of manganese superoxide dismutase in sporadic amyotrophic lateral sclerosis. Acta Neuropathol 1994; 88 (2): 151–8.

Wiedau-Pazos M., Goto J.J., Rabizadeh S., Gralla E.B., et al. Altered reactivity of superoxide dismutase in familial amyotrophic lateral sclerosis. Science 1996 Jan 26; 271 (5248): 515–8.

Yasui M., Ota K., Garruto R.M. Concentrations of zinc and iron in the brains of Guamanian patients with amyotrophic lateral sclerosis and parkinsonism-dementia. NeuroToxicology 1993 Winter; 14 (4): 445–50.

Yasui M., Yase Y., Kihira T., Adachi K., Suzuki Y. Magnesium and calcium contents in CNS tissues of amyotrophic lateral sclerosis patients from the Kii Peninsula, Japan. Eur Neurol 1992; 32: 95–8.

Yasui M., Yase Y., Ota K., Garruto R.M. Aluminum deposition in the central nervous system of patients with amyotrophic lateral sclerosis from the Kii Peninsula of Japan. NeuroToxicology 1991 Fall; 12 (3): 615–20.

Yasui M., Yase Y., Ota K., Mukoyama M., Adachi K. High aluminum deposition in the central nervous system of patients with amyotrophic lateral sclerosis from the Kii Peninsula, Japan: two case reports. NeuroToxicology 1991 Summer; 12 (2): 277–83.

Yee S. and Choi B.H. Oxidative stress in neurotoxic effects of methylmercury poisoning. NeuroToxicology 1996; 17 (1): 17–26.

Yim M.B., Kang J.H., Yim H.S., Kwak H.S., et al. A gain-of-function of an amyotrophic lateral sclerosis–associated Cu, Zn-superoxide dismutase mutant: an enhancement of free radical formation due to a decrease in Km for hydrogen peroxide. Proc Natl Acad Sci 1996 Jun 11; 93 (12): 5709–14.

Yoshida S., Mitani K., Wakayma I., Kihira T., Yase Y. Bunina body formation in amyotrophic lateral sclerosis: a morphometric-statistical and trace element study featuring aluminum. J Neurol Sci 1995 May; 130 (1): 88–94.

• *Chapter Nine: Attention Deficit Hyperactivity Disorder*

American Psychiatric Association Diagnostic and Statistic Manual of Mental Disorders 3rd Ed., Revised (DSM3R). American Psychiatric Association, Washington, D.C., 1987.

Agostini C., Trojan S., Bellu R., Riva E., Giovannini M. The Neurodevelopmental quotient of healthy term infants at 4 months and feeding practice: the role of long-chain polyunsaturated fatty acids. Ped Res 1995 Aug; 38: 262–6.

Amaducci L., Angst J., Bech P., Benkert O., et al. Consensus conference on the methodology of clinical traits of "Nootropics," Pharmacopsychiatry 1990; 23: 171–5.

Arnsten A,F., Steer J.C., Hunt R.D. The contribution of alpha 2-noradrenergic mechanisms of prefrontal corticol cognitive function. Potential significance for attention-deficit hyperactivity disorder. Arch Gen Psychiatry 1996 May; 53 (5): 448–55.

Banfi S. and Dorigotti L. Experimental behavioral studies with oxiracetam on different types of chronic cerebral impairment. Clin Neuropharmacol 1986; 9 Suppl: 19–26.

Bekaroglu M., Aslan Y., Gedik Y., Deger O., et al. Relationships between serum free fatty acids and zinc, and attention deficit hyperactivity disorder: a research note. J. Child Psychol. Psychiatry 1996 Fed; 37 (2): 225–7.

Benson D.F. The role of frontal dysfunction in attention deficit hyperactivity disorders. J of Child Neurol 1991; 6: 9–12.

Berry C., et al. Girls with attention deficit disorder, a silent minority? A report on behavioral and cognitive characteristics. Pediatrics 1985; 76: 801–9.

Boris M. and Mandel F.S. Foods and additives are common causes of the attention deficit hyperactive disorder in children. Ann Allergy 1994 May; 72 (5): 462–8.

Carter C.M., Urbanowicz M., Hemsley R., Mantilla L., et al. Effects of a few food diet in attention deficit disorder. Arch Dis Child 1993 Nov; 69 (5): 564–8.

Chopin P. and Briley M. Effects of four non-cholinergic cognitive enhancers in comparison with tacrine and galantamine on scopolamine-induced amnesia in rats. Psychopharmacology 1992; 106: 26–30.

Colburn T., Dumanosky D., and Myers J.P. Our Stolen Future. Penguin 1991; 185–9.

Egger J., Carter C.M., Graham P.J., Gumley D., Soothill J.F. Controlled trial of oligoantigenic treatment in the hyperkinetic syndrome. Lancet 1985 Mar 9: 540–5.

Egger J., Stolla A., McEwen L.M. Controlled trial of hyposensitization in children with food-induced hyperkinetic syndrome. Lancet 1992 May 9; 339: 1150–3.

Eisenberg J., Asnis G.M., van Praag H.M., Vela R.M. Effects of tyrosine on attention deficit order with hyperactivity. J Clin Psychiatry 1988 May; 49 (5): 193–5.

Eppright T.D., Sanfacon J.A., Horwitz E.A. Attention deficit hyperactivity disorder, infantile autism, and elevated blood-lead: a possible relationship. Mo Med 1996 Mar; 93 (3): 136–8.

Ernst M. and Zametkin A. The interface of genetics, neuroimaging and neurochemistry in attention deficit disorder. In Psychopharmacology, Fourth Generation of Progress. Blum F.E. and Kupfer D.J., eds. Raven Press, 1995.

Feingold, B. Why Your Child is Hyperactive. Random House, 1975.

Feingold, B. Hyperkinesis and learning disabilities linked to the ingestion of artificial food colors and flavors. J Learn Disabil 1976 (9): 551–59.

Findling R.L., Schwartz M.A., Flannery D.J., Manos M.J. Venlafaxine in adults with attention-deficit/hyperactivity disorder: an open clinical trial. J Clin Psychiatry 1996 May; 57 (5): 184–9.

Funk K.F. and Schmidt J. Effect of nootropics on choline uptake. Biomed Biochim Acta 1988; 47: 417–21.

Gibson R.A., Neumann M.A., Makrides M. Effect of dietary docosahexaenoic acid on brain composition and neural function in term infants. Lipids 1996; 31: S177–S93.

Girardi N.L., Shaywitz S.E., Shaywitz B.A., Marchione K., et al. Blunted catecholamine responses after glucose ingestion in children with attention deficit disorder. Ped Res 1995 Oct; 38 (4): 539–42.

Golub M.S., Keen C.L., Gershwin M.E., Hendrickx A.G. Developmental zinc deficiency and behavior. J Ntr 1995; 125: 2263S–2271S.

Gouliaev A.H. and Senning A. Piracetam and other structurally related nootropics. Brain Res Rev 1994; 19: 180–22.

Grau M., Montero J.L., Balasch J. Effect of piracetam on electrocortigram and local cerebral glucose utilization in the rat. Gen Pharmacol 1987; 18: 207–11.

Guilarte T.R., Miceli R.C., Jett D.A. Biochemical evidence of an interaction of lead at the zinc allosteric sites of the NMDA receptor complex: effects of neuronal development. NeuroToxicology 1995; 16 (1): 63–72.

Hauser P. Attention deficit hyperactivity disorder in people with generalized resistance to thyroid hormone. N Engl J Med 1993; 328: 997–1001.

Hjorther A., Browne E., Jkobsen K., et al. Organic brain syndrome treated with oxiracetam. A double-blind randomized controlled trial. Acta Neurol Scand 1987; 75: 271–6.

Joffe R.T. and Sokolov S.T.H. Thyroid hormones, the brain, and affective disorders. Critical Rev in Neurobiol 1994; 8(½): 46–53.

Kahn C.A., Kelly P.C., Walker W.O. Lead screening in children with attention deficit hyperactivity disorder and developmental delay. Clin Pediatr 1995 Sept; 34 (9): 498–501.

Kaneko M., et al. Hypothalamic-pituitary-adrenal axis function in children with attention deficit hyperactivity disorder. J Autism Dev Disord 1993 Mar; 23 (1): 59–65.

Lecaillon J.B., Dubois J.P., Coppens H., et al. Pharmacokinetics of oxiracetam in elderly patients after 800 mg oral doses, comparison with non-geriatric healthy subjects. Eur J Drug Metab Pharmacokinet, 1990; 15: 223–30.

Lenegre A., Chermat R., Avril I., et al. Specificity of piracetam's anti-amnesic activity in three models of amnesia in the mouse. Pharmacol Biochem Behav 1988; 29: 626–9.

Marret S., Gressens P., Gadisseux J.F., Evrard P. Prevention by magnesium of excitotoxic neuronal death in the developing brain: an animal model for clinical intervention studies. Dev Med Child Neurol 1995 Jun; 37 (6): 473–84.

McConnell H. Catecholamine metabolism in the attention deficit disorder: implications for the use of amino acid precursor therapy. Med Hypotheses 1985 Aug; 17 (4): 305–11.

Mefforid I.N. et al. A neuroanatomical and biochemical basis for attention deficit disorder with hyperactivity in children. A defect in tonic adrenal mediated inhibition of locus ceruleus stimulation. Med Hypotheses 1989; 29: 33–42.

Michals K. and Matalon R. Phenylalanine metabolites, attention span and hyperactivity. Am J Clin Nutr 1985 Aug; 42 (2): 361–5.

Mitchell E.A., Aman M.G., Turbott S.H. Clinical characteristics and serum essential fatty acid levels in hyperactive children. Clin Pediatr 1987 Aug; 26 (8): 406–11.

Needleman H.L., Riess JA., Tobin M.J., et al. Bone lead levels and delinquent behavior. JAMA 1996 Feb 7; 275 (5): 363–9.

Oades R.D. Attention deficit disorder with hyperactivity. The contribution of catecholinergic activity. Prog in Neurobiol 1987; 29: 365–91.

Piercey M.F., Vogelsang G.D., Franklin S.R., Tang A. H. Reversal of scopolamine-induced amnesia and alterations in energy metabolism by the nootropic piracetam: implications regarding identification of brain structures involved in consolidation of memory traces. Brain Res 1987; 424: 1–9.

Pliszka S.R., Hatch J.P., Borcherding S.H., Rogeness G.A. Classical conditioning in children with attention deficit hyperactivity disorder (ADHD) and anxiety disorders: a test of Quay's model. J abnorm Child Psychol 1993 Aug; 21 (4): 411–23.

Refetoff S., Weiss R.E., Usala S.J. The syndromes of resistance to thyroid hormone. Endocrine Rev 1993; 14 (3): 348–90.

Reimherr F.W., Wender P.H., Wood D.R., Ward M. An open trial of L-tyrosine in the treatment of attention deficit disorder, residual type. Am J Psychiatry 1987 Aug; 144 (8): 1071–3.

Rowe K.S. Synthetic food colourings and "hyperactivity": a double-blind crossover study. Aust Ped J 1988 Apr; 24 (2): 143–7.

Shanaz M.T. and Yang J. A time course of altered thyroid states on the noradrenergic system in rat brain by quantitative autoradiography. Neuroendocrinology 1994; 59: 235–44.

Shekim W.O., Antun F., Hanna G.L., McCracken J.T., Hess E.B. S-adenosyl-l-methionine (SAM) in adults with ADHD. Psychopharmacol Bull 1990; 26 (2): 249–53.

Stevens L.J., Zentall S.S., Deck J.L., Abate M.L., et al. Essential fatty acid metabolism in boys with attention deficit hyperactivity disorder. Am J Clin Nutr 1995 Oct; 62 (4): 761–8.

Tuthill, R.W. Hair lead levels related to children's classroom attention-deficit behavior. Arch Environ Health 1996 May-Jun; 51 (3): 214–20.

Tritschler H.J., Packer L., Medori R. Oxidative stress and mitochondrial dysfunction in neurodegeneration. Biochem Mol Biol Int 1994 Aug; 34 (1): 169–81.

Uauy R., Peirano P., Hoffman D., Mena P., Birch D., Birch E. Role of essential fatty acids in the function of the developing nervous system. Lipids 1996; 31: Supplement.

Ward N.I., et al. The influence of the chemical additive tartrazine on the zinc status of hyperactive children—a double-blind placebo-controlled study. J of Nutr Med 1990; 1: 51–57.

Weiss R.E., Stein M.A., Trommer B., Refetoff, S. Attention-deficit hyperactivity disorder and thyroid function. J Ped 1993 Oct; 123 (4): 539–45.

Wender E.H. and Solanto M.V. Effects of sugar on aggressive and inattentive behavior in children with attention deficit disorder with hyperactivity and normal children. Pediatrics 1991 Nov; 88 (5): 960–6.

Wilens T.E., Biederman J., Spencer T.J., Prince J. Pharmacotherapy of adult attention deficit/hyperactivity disorder: a review. J Clin Psycopharmacol 1995; 15 (4): 270–8.

Williams L.R. Oxidative stress, age-related neurodegeneration, and the potential for neurotrophic treatment. Cerebrovas Brain Metab Rev 1995 Spring; 7 (1): 55–73.

Wood D.R., Reimherr F.W., Wender P.H. Treatment of attention deficit disorder with DL-phenylalanine. Psychiatry Res 1985 Sept; 16 (1): 21–6.

Zametkin, Alan J. Cerebral glucose metabolism in adults with hyperactivity of childhood onset. N Engl J Med 1990 Nov 15; 323 (20): 1361–6.

## • Chapter Ten: Chronic Fatigue Syndrome

Amarakoon A.M., Tappia P.S., Grimble R.F. Endotoxin induced production of interleukin-6 is enhanced by vitamin E deficiency and reduced by black tea extract. Inflamm Res 1995 Jul; 44 (7): 301–5.

Araki R., Inoue S., Osborne M.P., Telang W. T. Chemoprevention of mammary preneoplasia. In vitro effects of a green tea polyphenol. Ann NY Acad Sci 1995; 768: 215–22.

Arora D. and Ross A.C. Antibody response against tetanus toxoid is enhanced by lipopolysaccharide or tumor necrosis factor-alpha in vitamin A-sufficient and deficient rats. Am J Clin Nutr 1994; 59 (4): 922–8.

Barnes P.R., Taylor D.J., Kemp G.J., Radda G.K. Skeletal muscle bioenergetics in the chronic fatigue syndrome. J Neurol Neurosurg Psychiatry 1993 Jun; 56 (6): 679–83.

Baum C.G., Szabo P., Siskind G.W., et al. Cellular control of IGE induction by a polyphenol-rich compound. Preferential activation of TH2 cells. J Immunol 1990; 145 (3): 779–84.

Behan P.O., Haniffah A.G., Doogan D.P., Loudon M. A pilot study of sertraline for the treatment of chronic fatigue syndrome. Ann Int Med 1992 Nov; 117 (10): 854–63.

Behan W.M. and Behan P.O. The role of viral infection in polymyositis dermatomyositis and chronic fatgue syndrome. Clin Neurol 1993 Nov; 2 (3): 637–57.

Bell S.J., Chavali S., Bistrian B.R., et al. Dietary fish oil and cytokine and eicosanoid production during human immunodeficiency virus infection. J Parenter Enteral Nutr 1996 Jan-Feb; 20 (1): 43–9.

Benfield T.L., van Steenwijk R., Nielsen T.L., et al. Interleukin-8 and eicosanoid production in the lung during moderate to severe Pneumocystis carinii pneumonia in AIDS: a role of interleukin-8 in the pathogenesis of P. carinii pneumonia. Respir Med 1995 Apr; 89 (4): 285–90.

Blomhoff H.K., et al. Vitamin A is a key regulator for cell growth, cytokine production, and differentiation in normal B cells. J Biol Chem 1992; 267 (33): 23988–92.

Bou-Holaigah I., Rowe P.C., Kan J., Calkins H. The relationship between neurally mediated hypotension and the chronic fatigue syndrome. JAMA 1995 Sept 27; 274 (12): 961–7.

Bowles N.E., Bayston T.A., Zhang H.Y., Dowyl D., et al. Persistance of enterovirus RNA in muscle biopsy samples suggest that some cases of chronic fatigue syndrome result from a previous, inflammatory viral myopathy. J Med 1993; 24 (2–3): 145–60.

Brechel M.M., Lozano Y., Wright M.A., et al. Immune modulation by interleukin-12 in tumor-bearing mice receiving vitamin D3 treatments to block induction of immunosuppressive granulocyte/macrophage progenitor cells. Cancer Immunol Immunother 1996 May; 42 (4): 213–20.

Brohee D. and Neve P. Effect of dietary high doses of vitamin E on the cell size of T and B lymphocyte subsets in young and old CBA mice. Mech Aging Dev 1995 Nov 24; 85 (2–3): 147–55.

Buchwald D., Cheney P.R., Peterson D.L., Henry B., et al. A chronic illness characterized by fatigue, neurologic and immunologic disorders, and active human herpesvirus type 6 infection. Ann Int Med 1992 Jan; 116 (2): 103–13.

Buffi O., Ciaroni S., Guidi L., Cecchini T., Bombardelli E. Morphological analysis on the adrenal zona fasciculata of Ginseng, Ginsenoside Rb1 and Geinsenoside Rg1 treated mice. Boll Soc Ital Biol Sper 1993 Dec; 69 (12): 791–7.

Bukovsky M., et al. Immunomodulating activity of echinacea gloriosa L., echinacea angustifolia DC. and rudbeckia speciosa Wenderoth ethanol-water extracts. J Pharmacol 1995 Mar-Apr; 47 (2): 175–7.

Bukovsky M., Vaverkova S., Kostalova D., Magnusova R. Immunomodulating activity of ethanol-water extracts of the roots of echinacea gloriosa L., echinacea angustifolia D.C. and rudbeckia speciosa Wenderoth tested on the immune system in C57BL6 inbred mice. Cesk Farm 1993 Aug; 42 (4): 184–7.

Calabrese L.H., Danao T., Camara E.G., Wilde W.S. Chronic fatigue and immune dysfunction. Cleve Clin J Med 1992 Mar-Apr; 59 (2): 123–4.

Carrick J.B., Schnellmann R.G., Moore J.N. Dietary source of omega-3 fatty acids affects endotoxin-induced peritoneal macrophage tumor necrosis factor and eicosanoid synthesis. Shock 1994; 2 (6): 421–6.

Carver J.D. Dietary nucleotides: cellular immune, intestinal and hepatic system effects. J Nutr 1994; 124: 144S–146S.

Chung F.L., XU Y., Ho C.T., Han C. Possible mechanism of inhibition of tobacco-specific nitrosamine-induced lung tumorigenesis in A/J mice by green tea and its polyphenol. Proc Ann Meet Am Assoc Cancer Res 1992; 33: A962.

Clague J.E., et al. Intravenous magnesium loading and chronic fatigue syndrome. Lancet 1992 Jul 11; 340: 124–5.

Cox I.M., et al. Red blood cell magnesium and chronic fatigue syndrome. Lancet 1991 Mar 30; 337 (8744): 757–60.

Coyle P.K., Krupp L.B., Doscher C., Amin K. Borrelia burgdorferi reactivity in patients with severe persistent fatigue who are from a region in which Lyme disease is endemic. Clin Infectious Disease 1994; 18 (Suppl 1): 24–7.

De Caterina R., Cybulsky M.I., Clinton S.K., et al. The omega-3 fatty acid docosahexaenoate reduces cytokine-induced expression of proatherogenic and proinflammatory proteins in human endothelial cells. Arterioscler Thromb 1994; 14 (11): 1829–36.

Demitrack, M.A. Chronic fatigue syndrome: a disease of the hypothalamic-pituitary-adrenal axis? Ann Med 1994 Feb; 26 (1): 1–5.

Demitrack M.A., et al. Evidence for impaired activation of the hypothalamic pituitary-adrenal axis in patients with chronic fatigue syndrome. J Clin Endocrinology and Metabolis 1991; 73: 1224–34.

de Vries H.E., Hoogendoorn K.H., van Dijk J., et al. Eicosanoid production by rat cerebral endothelial cells: stimulation by lipopolysaccharide, interleukin-1 and interleukin-6. J Neuroimmunol 1995 Jun; 59 (1–2): 1–8.

Dorsch W. Clinical application of extracts of echinacea purpurea or echinacea pallida. Z Arztl Fortbild 1996 Apr; 90 (2): 117–22.

Fujibayashi S., Suzuki S., Okano K., Naitoh T., et al. The weak calcemic vitamin D3 analogue 22-oxacalcitriol suppresses the production of tumor necrosis factor-alpha by peripheral mononuclear cells. Immunol Lett 1991; 30 (3): 307–11.

Fukui H., Goto K., Tabata M. Two antimicrobial flavanones from the leaves of glycyrrhiza glabra. Chem Pharm Bull 1988 Oct; 36 (10): 4174.

Goldenberg D.L. Fibromyalgia and its relation to chronic fatigue syndrome, viral illness and immune abnormalities. J Rheumatol 1989 Nov; 19: (Suppl) 91–3.

Gray J.B. and Martinovic A.M. Eicosanoids and essential fatty acid modulation in chronic disease and the chronic fatigue syndrome. Med Hypotheses 1994 Jul; 43 (1): 31–42.

Guo Q., Peng T.Q., Yang Y.Z. Effect of Astragalus membranaceous on Ca2+ influx and coxsackie virus B3 RNA replication in cultured neonatal rat heart cells. Chung Kuo Chung Hsi I Chieh Ho Tsa Chih 1995 Aug; 15 (8): 483–5.

Haverty T., Haddad J.G., Neilson E.G. 1,25-dihydroxyvitamin D3 stimulates interleukin-2 production by a T cell lymphoma line (MLA-144) cultured in vitamin D-deficient rat serum. J Leukoc Biol 1987 Feb; 41 (2): 177–82.

Hiai S., Sasayama Y., Oguro C. Chronic effects of ginseng saponin, glycyrrhizin and flavin adenine dinucleotide on adrenal and thymus weight in normal and dexamethasone-treated rats. Chem Pharm Bull 1987 Jan; 35 (1): 241–8.

Hibino Y., Konishi Y., Koike J., Tabata T., et al. Productions of interferon-gamma and nitrite are induced in mouse splenic cells by a heteroglycan-protein fraction from culture medium of Lentinus edodes mycelia. Immunopharmacol 1994 Jul-Aug; 28 (1): 77–85.

Hilgers A. and Frank J. Chronic fatigue syndrome: immune dysfunction, role of pathogens and toxic agents and neurological and cardial changes. Wien Med Wochenschr 1994; 144 (16): 399–406.

Hirata A., Adachi Y., Itoh W., et al. Monoclonal antibody to proteoglycan derived from grifola frondosa (maitake) Biol Pharm Bull 1994 Apr; 17 (4): 539–42.

Hishida I., Nanba H., Kuroda H. Antitumor activity exhibited by orally administered extract from fruit body of grifola frondosa (maitake). Chem Pharm Bull 1988; 36 (5): 1819–27.

Howard J.M., et al. Magnesium and chronic fatigue syndrome. Lancet 1992 Aug 15; 340: 426.

Huang Z., Quin N.P., Ye W. Effect of astragalus membranaceous on T-lymphocyte subsets in patients with viral myocarditis. Chung Kuo Chung Hsi I Chieh Ho Tsa Chih 1995 Jun; 15 (6): 328–30.

Jones J.F., Streib J., Baker S., Herberger M. Chronic fatigue syndrome: I. Epstein-Barr virus immune response and molecular epidemiology. J Med Virol 1991 Mar; 33 (3): 151–8.

Ju H.S., Li X.J., Zaho B.L., et al. Effects of glycyrrhiza flavonoid on lipid peroxidation and active oxygen radicals. Yao Hsueh Pao 1989; 24 (11): 807–12.

Jyonouchi H. Nucleotide actions on humoral immune responses. J Nutr 1994; 124: 138S–140S.

Katiyar S.K., Agarwal R., Mukhtar H. Inhibition of both stage I and stage II skin tumor promotion in SENCAR mice by a polyphenolic fraction isolated from green tea: inhibition depends on the duration of polyphenol treatment. Carcinogenesis 1993; 14 (12): 2641–3.

Keller R.H., Lane J.L., Klimas N., Reiter W.M., et al. Association between HLA class II antigens and the chronic fatigue immune dysfunction syndrome. Clin Infect Dis 1994 Jan; 18 (Suppl 1): S154–6.

Kent-Braun J.A., Sharma K.R., Weiner M.W., Massie B., Miller R.G. Central basis of muscle fatigue in chronic fatigue syndrome. Neurol 1993 Sept; 43 (9): 1866–7.

Komaroff A.L. Chronic fatigue syndromes: relationship to chronic viral infections. J Virol Methods 1988 Sept; 21 (1–4): 3–10.

Kramer T.R., Udomkesmalee E., Dhanamitta S., et al. Lymphocyte responsiveness of children supplemented with vitamin A and zinc. Am J Clin Nutr 1993 Oct; 58 (4): 566–70.

Kulkarni A.D., Rudolph F.B., Van Buren C.T. The role of dietary sources of nucleotides in immune function: a review. American Institute of Nutrition 1994.

Kuratsune H., Yamaguti K., Takahashi M., et al. Acetylcarnitine deficiency in chronic fatigue syndrome. Clin Infectious Diseases 1994; 18 (Suppl 1): S62–7.

Land J.M., Kemp G.J., Taylor D.J., Standing S.J., et al. Oral phosphate supplements reverse skeletal muscle abnormalities in a case of chronic fatigue with idiopathic renal hypophosphatemia. Neuromuscul Disord 1993 May; 3 (3): 223–5.

Lei L.S. and Lin Z.B. Effects of ganoderma polysaccharides on the activity of DNA polymerase alpha of splenocytes and immune function in aged mice. Yao Hsueh Hsueh Pao 1993; 28 (8): 577–82.

Levy J.A. Viral studies of chronic fatigue syndrome. Clin Infect Dis 1994 Jan; 18 (Suppl 1): S1117–20.

Liang H., Wang Z., Tian F., Geng B. Effects of astragalus polysaccharides and ginsenoisides of ginseng stems and leaves on lymphocytes membrane fluidity and lipid peroxidation in traumatized mice. Chung Kuo Chung Yao Tsa Chih 1995 Sept; 20 (9): 558–60.

Lin J.M., et al. Evaluation of the anti-inflammatory and liver-protective effects of anoectochilus formosanus, ganoderma lucidum and gynostemma pentaphyllum in rats. Am J Chin Med 1993; 21 (1): 59–69.

Lloyd A.R. and Klimas N. Summary: immunologic studies of chronic fatigue syndrome. Clin Infectious Diseases 1994; 18 (Suppl 1): S160–1.

Lu Z.W. Psychoneuroimmunological effects of morphine and the immunoprotection of ganoderma polysaccharides peptide in morphine-dependent mice. Sheng Li Ko Hsueh Chin Chan 1995 Jan; 26 (1): 45–9.

Manu P., Matthews D.A., Lane T.J. Food intolerance in patients with chronic fatigue. Int J Eat Disord 1993 Mar; 13 (2): 203–9.

McCully K.K., Natelson B.H., Iotti S., Sisto S., Leigh J.S. Reduced oxidative muscle metabolism in chronic fatigue syndrome. Muscle Nerve 1996 May; 19 (5): 621–5.

Meydani S.N. Interaction of omega-3 polyunsaturated fatty acids and vitamin E on the immune response. World Rev Nutr Diet 1994; 75: 155–61.

Muller-Jakic B., Brew W., Probstle A., Redl K., et al. In vitro inhibition of cyclooxygenase and 5-lipoxygenase by alkamides from echinacea and achillea species. Planta Med 1994 Feb; 60 (1): 37–40.

Nanba H. Activity of maitake D-fraction to inhibit carcinogenesis and metastasis. Ann NY Acad Sci 1995 Sept 30; 768: 243–5.

Ojo-Amaize E.A., Conley E.J., Peter J.B. Decreased natural killer cell activity is associated with severity of chronic fatigue immune dysfunction syndrome. Clin Infect Dis 1994 Jan; 18 (Suppl 1): S157–9.

Okano M. Viral infection and its causative role for chronic fatigue syndrome. Nippon Rinsho 1992 Nov; 50 (11): 2617–24.

Oxholm A., Oxholm P., Staberg B., Bendtzen K. Expression of interleukin-6-like molecules and tumor necrosis factor after topical treatment of psoriasis with a new vitamin D analogue (MC 903). Acta Derm Venereol 1989; 69 (5): 385–90.

Patarca R., Klimas N.G., Lugtendorf S., Antoni M., Fletcher M.A. Dysregulated expression of tumor necrosis factor in chronic fatigue syndrome: interrelations with cellular sources and patterns of soluble immune mediator expression. Clin Infect Dis 1994 Jan; 18 (Suppl 1): S147–53.

Plioplys A.V. and Plioplys S. Electron-microscopic investigation of muscle mitochondria in chronic fatigue syndrome. Neuropsychobiology 1995; 32 (4): 175–81.

Potaznick W. and Kozol N. Ocular manifestations of chronic fatigue and immune dysfunction syndrome. Optom Vis Sci 1992 Oct; 69 (10): 811–4.

Rosen P. The synergism of gamma-interferon and tumor necrosis factor in whole body hypothermia with vitamin C to control toxicity. Med Hypotheses 1992; 38 (3): 257–8.

Rowe P.C., Bou-Holaigah I., Flynn J., Kan J., Calkins H. Information for physicians. The Johns Hopkins Hospital, 1995 Oct.

Sakamotol K., Reddy D., Hara Y., Milner J.A. Impact of green or black tea polyphenol on canine mammary tumor cells in culture. Proc Annu Meet Am Assoc Cancer Res 1995; 36: A3542.

Sandman C.A., Barron J.L., Nackoul K., et. al. Memory deficits associated with chronic fatigue immune dysfunction syndrome. Biol Psychiatry 1993 Apr 15-May 1; 33 (8–9): 618–23.

Sarkar S., Koga J., Whitley R.J., Chatterjee S. Antiviral effect of the extract of culture medium of Lentinus edodes mycelia on the replication of herpes simplex virus type 1. Antiviral Res 1993 Apr; 20 (4): 293–303.

Shimizu N., Tomoda M., Takada K., Gonda R. The core structure and immunological activities of glycyrrhizin UA, the main polysaccharide from the root of glycyrrhiza uralensis. Chem Pharm Bull 1992 Aug: (40*8): 2125–8.

Stabel J.R. and Goff J.P. Influence of vitamin D3 infusion and dietary calcium on secretion of interleukin 1, interleukin 6, and tumor necrosis factor in mice infected with Mycobacterium paratuberculosis. Am J Vet Res 1996 Jun; 57 (6): 825–9.

Steinmuller C., Roesler J., Grottrup E., et al. Polysaccharides isolated from plant cell cultures of echinacea purpurea enhance the resistance if immunosuppressed mice against systemic infections with candida albicans and Listeria monocytogenes. Int J Immunopharmacol 1993 Jul; 15 (5): 605–14.

Sternberg E., Chrouusos G.P., Wilder R.L., Gold P.W. The stress response and the regulation of inflammatory disease. Ann Internal Med 1992 Nov 15; 117 (10): 854–66.

Sugiura H., Nichida H., Inaba R., Iwata H. Effects of exercise in the growing stage in mice and of astragalus membranaceous on immune functions. Nipon Eiseigaku Zasshi 1993 Feb; 47 (6): 1021–31.

Suzuki I., Hashimoto K., Oikawa S., Sato K., et al. Antitumor and immunomodulating activities of a beta-glucan obtained from liquid-cultured grifola frondosa. Chem Pharm Bull 1989; 37 (2): 410–13.

Swartz M.N. N Engl J Med 1988 Dec 29; 319 (26): 1726–8.

Tachikawa E., Kudo K., Kashimoto T., Takahashi E. Ginseng saponins reduced acetylcholine-evoked Na+ influx and catecholamine secretion in bovine adrenal chromaffin cells. J Pharmacol Exp Ther 1995 May; 273 (2): 629–36.

Taimi M., Defacque H., Commes T., et al. Effect of retinoic acid and vitamin D on the expression of interleukin-6 in the human monocytic cell line U937. Immunology 1993 Jun; 79 (2): 229–35.

Takahashi H., Imai K., Katanuma A., Sugaya T., et al. A case of chronic fatigue syndrome who showed a beneficial effect by intravenous administration of magnesium sulphate. Arerugi 1992 Nov; 41 (11): 1605–10.

Takeyama T., et al. Host-mediated antitumor effect of grifolan NMF-5N, a polysaccharide obtained from grifola frondosa. J Pharmacobiodyn 1987; 10 (11): 644–51.

Takeyama T., et al. Vitamin E increases interleukin-2 dependent cellular growth and glycoprotein glycosylation in murine cytotoxic T-cell line. Biochem Biophy Res Commun 1993 Jun 30; 193 (3): 872–7.

Telang N.T., Inoue S., Bradlow H.L., Fujiki H., Osborne M.P. Antipromotional effect of a green tea polyphenol on c-myc-transfected mammary epithelial cells. Proc Annu Meet Am Assoc Cancer Res 1994; 35: A3692.

Uchida A. Chronic fatigue immune dysfunction syndrome. Nippon Rinsho 1992 Nov; 50 (11): 2625–9.

Walker W.A. Nucleotides and nutrition: role as dietary supplement. J Nutr 1994; 124: 121S–123S.

Wang Y., Huang D.S., Eskelson C.D., Watson R.R. Long-term dietary vitamin E retards development of retrovirus-induced disregulation in cytokine production. Clin Immunol Immunopathol 1994; 72 (1): 70–5.

Wang Y., Huang D.S., Watson R.R. Dietary vitamin E modulation of cytokine production by splenocytes and thymocytes from alcohol-fed mice. Alcohol Clin Exp Res 1994; 18 (2): 355–62.

Wang Y., Huang D.S., Watson R.R. Vitamin E supplementation modulates cytokine production by thymocytes during murine AIDS. Immunol Res 1993; 12 (4): 358–66.

Wang Y. and Watson R.R. Vitamin E supplementation at various levels alters cytokine production by thymocytes during retrovirus infection causing murine AIDS. Thymus 1994; 22 (3): 153–65.

Weng X.S. Treatment of leucopenia with pure astragalus preparation—an analysis of 115 leukocopenic cases. Chung Kuo Chung Hsi I Chieh Ho Tsa Chih 1995; 15 (8): 462–4.

Wong R., Lopaschuk G., Zhu G., Walker D., et al. Skeletal muscle metabolism in the chronic fatigue syndrome. Chest 1992 Dec; 102 (6): 1716–22.

Xu Y., Ho C.T., Amin S.G., Han C., Chung F.L. Inhibition of tobacco-specific nitrosamine-induced lung tumorigenesis in A/J mice by green tea and its major polyphenol as antioxidants. Cancer Res 1992; 52 (14): 3875–9.

Yamashiki M., Nichimura A., Kosaka Y. Effects of methylcobalamin (vitamin B12) on in vitro cytokine production of peripheral blood mononuclear cells. J Clin Lab Immunol 1992; 37 (4): 173–82.

Yang G. and Yu Y. Immunopotentiating effect of traditional Chinese drugs—ginsenoside and glycyrrhiza polysaccharide. Porc Chin Acad Med Sci Peking Union Med Coll 1990; 5 (4): 188–93.

Yu W., Sanders B.G., Kline K. Modulation of murine EL-4 thymic lymphoma cell proliferation any cytokine production by vitamin E succinate. Nutr Cancer 1996; 25 (2): 137–49.

Zhang L.X., Mong H., Zhou X.B. Effect of Japanese ganoderma lucidum on production of interleukin-2 from murine splenocytes. Chung Kuo Chung Hsi I Chieh Ho Tsa Chih 1993 Oct; 13 (10): 613–15.

Zhao T.H. Positive modulating action of shengmaisan with astragalus membranaceous on anti-tumor activity of LAK cells. Chung Kuo Chung Hsi I Chieh Ho Tsa Chih 1993 Aug; 13 (8): 471–2.

## • Chapter Eleven: Depression

Abou-Saleh M.T. and Coppen A. The biology of folate in depression: implications for nutritional hypotheses of the psychoses. J Psychiatr Res 1986; 20 (2): 91–101.

Abou-Saleh M.T. and Coppen A. Serum and red blood cell folate in depression. Acta Psychiatr Scand 1989 Jul; 80 (1): 78–82.

Altamura C., Maes M., Dai J., Meltzer H.Y. Plasma concentrations of excitatory amino acids, serine, glycine, taurine and histidine in major depression. Eur Neuropsychopharmacol 1995; 5 (Suppl): 71–5.

Amato L., Paolisso G., Cacciatore F., Ferrara N., et al. Non-insulin-dependent diabetes mellitus is associated with a greater prevalence of depression in the elderly. Diabetes Metab 1996 Oct; 22 (5): 314–8.

Anderson I.M., Parry-Billings M., Newsholme E.A., Poortmans J.R., Cowen P.J. Decreased plasma tryptophan concentration in major depression: relationship to melancholia and weight loss. J Affect Disord 1990 Nov; 20 (3): 185–91.

Bell I.R., Edman J.S., Morrow F.D., Marby D.W., et al. B complex vitamin patterns in geriatric and young adult in patients with major depression. J Am Geriatr Soc 1991 Mar; 39 (3): 252–7.

Bell I.R., Edman J.S., Morrow F.D., Marby D.W., et al. Vitamin B1, B2, and B6 augmentation of tricyclic antidepressant treatment in geriatric depression with cognitive dysfunction. J Am Coll Nutr 1992 Apr; 11 (2): 159–63.

Bell K.M., Plon L., Bunney W.E., Potkin S.G. S-adenosylmethionine treatment of depression: a controlled clinical trial. Am J Psychiatry 1988 Sept; 145 (9): 1110–4.

Bladt S. and Wagner H. Inhibition of MAO by fractions and constituents of hypericum extract. J Geriatr Psychiatry Neurol 1994 Oct; 7 (Suppl 1): S57–9.

Bottiglieri T., Godfrey P., Flynn T., Carney M.W. et al. Cerebrospinal fluid S-adenosylmethionine in depression and dementia: effects of treatment with parenteral and oral S-adenosylmethionine. J Neurol Neurosurg Psychiatry 1990 Dec; 53 (12): 1096–8.

Bottiglieri T. and Hyland K. S-adenosylmethionine levels in psychiatric and neurological disorders: a review. Acta Neurol Scand 1994; Supplement 154: 19–26.

Bottiglieri T., Hyland K., Laundy M., Godfrey P., Carney M.W., Toone B.K., Reynolds E.H. Psychol Med 1992 Nov; 22(4): 871–6.

Candito M., Souetre E., Iordache A., Pringuey D., et al. Diurnal variation in total plasma tryptophan in controls and in depression. J Psychiatr Res 1990; 24 (3): 227–30.

Charles H.C., Lazeyras F., Krishnan K.R., Boyko O.B., et al. Brain choline in depression: in vivo detection of potential pharmacodynamic effects of antidepressant therapy using hydrogen localized spectroscopy. Prog Neuropsychopharmacol Biol Psychaitry 1994 Nov; 18 (7): 1121–7.

Coppen A., Swade C., Jones S.A., Armstrong R.A., Blair J.A., Leeming R.J. Depression and tetrahydrobiopterin: the folate connection. J Affect Disord 1989 Mar–Jun; 16 (2–3): 103–7.

Cowen P.J. and Charig E.M. Neuroendocrine responses to intravenous tryptophan in major depression. Arch Gen Psychiatry 1987 Nov; 44 (11): 958–66.

Delgado P.L., Charney C.S., Price L.H., et al. Neuroendocrine and behavioral effects of dietary tryptophan restriction in healthy subjects. Life Science 1990; 45: 2323–32.

Fava M. Rapidity of onset of the antidepressant effect of parenteral S-adenosyl L-methionine. Psych Res 1995; 956: 295–7.

Fuller R.W. The involvement of serotonin in regulation of pituitary adrenal cortical function. Frontiers of Neuroendocrinology 1992; 13: 250–70.

Gelenberg A.J., Wojcik J.D., Falk W.E., Baldessarini R.J., et al. Tyrosine for depression: a double-blind trial. J Affect Disord 1990 Jun; 19 (2): 125–32.

Haleem D.J., Yasmeen A., Haleem M.A., Zafar A. 24h withdrawal following repeated administration of caffeine attenuates brain serotonin but not tryptophan in rat brain: implications for caffeine-induced depression. Life Sci 1995; 57 (19): PL285–92.

Hansgen K.D., Vesper J., Ploch M. Multicenter double-blind study examining the antidepressant effectiveness of the hypericum extract LI 160. J Geriatr Psychiatry Neurol 1994 Oct; 7 (Suppl 1): 215–8.

Harrer G., Hubner W.D., Podzuweit H. Effectiveness and tolerance of the hypericum extract LI 160 compared to maprotiline: a multicenter double-blind study. J Geriatr Psychiatry Neurol 1994 Oct; 7 (Suppl 1): S24–8.

Harrer G. and Schulz V. Clinical investigation of the antidepressant effectiveness of hypericum. J Geriatr Psychiatry Neurol 1994 Oct; 7 (Suppl): S6–8.

Hibbeln J.R. and Salem N. Dietary polyunsaturated fatty acids and depression: when cholesterol does not satisfy. Am J Clin Nutr 1995; 62 (1): 1–9.

Hubner W.D., Lande S., Podzueweit H. Hypericum treatment of mild depressions with somatic symptoms. J Geriatr Psychiatry Neurol 1994 Oct; 7 (Suppl 1): S12–4.

Jeanningros R., Serres F., Dassa D., Azorin J.M., Grignon S. Red blood cell L-tryptophan uptake in depression: kinetic analysis in untreated depressed patients and healthy volunteers. Psychiatry Res 1996 Jul 31; 63 (2–3): 151–9.

Kagan B.L., Sultzer D.L., Rosenlicht N., Gerner R.H. Oral s-adenosylmethionine in depression: a randomized, double-blind, placebo-controlled trial. Am J Psychiatry 1990 May; 147 (5): 591–595.

Knapp S. and Irwin M. Plasma levels of tetrahydrobiopterin and folate in major depression. Biol Psychiatry 1989 Jun; 26 (2): 156–62.

Kofman O., Bersudsky U., Vinnitsky I., Alpert C., Belmaker R.H. The effect of peripheral inositol injection on rat motor activity models of depression. Isr J Med Sci 1993 Sept; 29 (9): 580–6.

Kumar A., Newberg A., Alavi A., Berlin J., et al. Regional cerebral glucose metabolism in late-life depression and Alzheimer's disease: a preliminary positron emission tomography study. Proc Natl Acad Sci 1993 Aug 1; 90 (15): 7019–23.

Levine J., Barak Y., Gonzalves M., Szor H., et al. Double-blind controlled trial of inositol treatment of depression. Am J Psychiatry 1995 May; 152 (5): 792–4.

Lopez J.F., Kathol R.G., Jaeckle R.S., Meller W. The HPA axis response to insulin hypoglycemia in depression. Biol Psychiatry 1987 Feb; 22 (2): 153–66.

Linde K., et al. St. John's wort for depression—an overview and meta-analysis of randomised clinical trials. BMJ 1996 Aug 3; 313 (7052): 253–8.

Maes M. and Meltzer H. The serotonin hypothesis of major depression. In Psychopharmacology, Fourth Generation of Progress, Blum F. and Kupfer B., eds. Raven Press, 1995.

Maes M., et al. The relationship between the viability of L-tryptophan to the brain. The spontaneous HPA axis activity and the HPA axis response to dexamethasone in depressed patients. Amino Acids 1991; 1: 57–65.

Maes M., et al. Suppressant effect of dexamethasone on the availability of plasma L-tryptophan and tyrosine in health control and in depressed patients. Acta Psychiatrica Scand 1990; 81: 19–23.

Maes M., Scharpe S., Meltzer H.Y., Okayli G., et al. Increased neopterin and interferon-gamma secretion and lower availability of L-tryptophan in major depression: further evidence for an immune response. Psychiatry Res 1994 Nov; 54 (2): 143–60.

Maes M., Meltzer H.Y., Scharpe S., Bosmans E., et al. Relationships between lower plasma L-tryptophan levels and immune-inflammatory variables in depression. Psychiatry Res 1993 Nov; 49 (2): 151–65.

Maes M., Smith R., Cristophe A., Cosyns P., et al. Fatty acid composition in major depression: decreased omega 3 fractions in cholesteryl esters and increased C20: 4 omega 6/C20:5 omega 3 ratio in cholesteryl esters and phospholipids. J Affect Disord 1996 Apr 26; 38 (1): 35–46.

Maes M., Wauters A., Verkerk R., Demedts P., et al. Lower serum L-tryptophan availability in depression as a marker of a more generalized disorder in protein metabolism. Neuropsychopharacology 1996 Sept; 15 (3): 243–51.

Martinez B., Kasper S., Ruhrmann S., Moller H.J. Hypericum in the treatment of seasonal affective disorders. J Geriatr Psychiatry Neurol 1994 Oct; 7 (Suppl 1): S29–33.

Maurizi C.P. The therapeutic potential for tryptophan and melatonin: possible roles in depression, sleep, Alzheimer's disease and abnormal aging. Med Hypotheses 1990 Mar; 31 (3): 233–42.

McCarty, M.F. Enhancing central and peripheral insulin activity as strategy for the treatment of endogenous depression—an adjuvant role for chromium picolinate? Med Hypotheses 1994 Oct; 43 (4): 247–52.

Moller S.E., et al. Plasma ratio tryptophan to neutral amino acids in relation to clinical response to paroxetine and clomipramine in patients with major depression. J Psychiatric Disord 1990; 18: 59–66.

Muller W.E. and Rossol R. Effects of hypericum extract on the expression of serotonin receptors. J Geriatr Psychiatry Neurol 1994 Oct; 7 (Suppl 1): S63–4.

Quintana J., et al. Platelet serotonin and plasma tryptophan decreases in endogenous depression. Clinical, therapeutic, and biological correlations. J Affect Disord 1992 Feb; 24 (2): 55–62.

Rasmussen H.H., Mortensen P.B., Jensen I.W. Depression and magnesium deficiency. Int J Psychiatry Med 1989; 19 (1): 57–63.

Rauch T.M. and Lieberman H.R. Tyrosine pretreatment reverses hypothermia-induced behavioral depression. Brain Res Bull 1990 Jan; 24 (1): 147–50.

Raucoules D., Azorin J.M., Barre A., Tissot R. Plasma levels and membrane transports in red blood cell of tyrosine and tryptophane in depression. Evaluation at baseline and recovery. Encephale 1991 May-Jun; 17 (3): 197–201.

Schiffer, R.B. Depressive syndromes associated with diseases of the central nervous system. Seminars in Neurology 1990 Sept; 10 (3): 239–44.

Schmidt U. and Sommer H. St. John's wort extract in the ambulatory therapy of depression. Attention and reaction ability are preserved. Fortschr Med 1993 Jul 10; 111 (19): 339–42.

Sommer H. and Harrer G. Placebo-controlled double-blind study examining the effectiveness of an hypericum preparation in 105 mildly depressed patients. J Geriatr Psychiatry Neurol 1994 Oct; 7 (Suppl 1): S9–11.

Van Praag H.M. In search of the mode of action of antidepressants: 5-HTP/tyrosine mixtures in depression. Adv Biochem Psychopharmacol 1984; 39: 301–14.

Vorbach E.U., Hubner W.D., Arnoldt K.H. Effectiveness and tolerance of the hypericum extract LI 160 in comparison with imipramine: randomized double-blind study with 135 outpatients, J Geriatr Psychiatry Neurol 1994 Oct; 7 (Suppl 1): S19–23.

Winokur A., Maislin G., Phillips J.L. Insulin resistance after oral glucose tolerance testing in patients with major depression. Am J Psychiatry 1988 Mar; 145 (3): 325–30.

Winokur A., Maislin G., Phillips J.L., Amsterdam J.D. Insulin resistance after oral glucose tolerance testing in patients with major depression. Am J Psychiatry 1988 Mar; 145 (3): 325–30.

Yamauchi A., Takei I., Kasuga A., Kitamura Y., et al. Depression of dehydroepiandrosterone in Japanese diabetic men—comparison between non-insulin-dependent diabetes mellitus and impaired glucose tolerance. Eur J Endocrinol 1996 Jul; 135 (1): 101–4.

Young S.N. Tryptophan depletion causes a rapid lowering of mood in normal males. Psychopharmacol 1985; 87: 173–7.

# INDEX

## ABOUT THE AUTHORS

DR. JAY LOMBARD is in private practice in neurology and neuropsychiatry, and employs traditional and complementary medical approaches in treating a wide spectrum of neurological and neuropsychiatric diseases. Formerly the chief resident of neurology at Long Island Jewish Medical Center, he is board certified by the American Board of Psychiatry and Neurology in neurology. Dr. Lombard is currently chief of neurology at Westchester Square Medical Center in the Bronx and voluntary staff attending at Albert Einstein College of Medicine Hospital. A member of the Medical Advisory Panel for the Cure Autism Now Foundation, he has lectured extensively on both the neurobiology of the autistic syndrome and on the application of complementary medicine in neurological diseases. In 1997, Dr. Lombard was named one of the best doctors in New York in *How to Find the Best Doctors in the New York Metro Area.*

CARL GERMANO, RD, CNS, LDN, is a registered certified nutritionist and practitioner in Chinese herbology. He holds a master's degree in clinical nutrition from New York University and has nearly twenty years of experience using innovative, complementary nutritional therapies in private clinical practice. For the past decade, he has dedicated his efforts to research and product development for the nutritional supplement industry, where he has been instrumental in bringing cutting-edge nutritional substances and formulas to the market. Presently, he is the Director of Product Development for Solgar Vitamin and Herb Company. Additionally, he is adjunct professor of nutrition at New York Chiropractic College and a frequent radio guest and columnist in nutrition.